THE CONSUMER HANDBOOK ON DIZZINESS AND VERTIGO

Dennis Poe, MD, Editor

Auricle Ink Publishers * Sedona Arizona

Library of Congress Cataloging-in-Publication Data
The consumer handbook on dizziness and vertigo /
by Dennis Poe.-- 1st ed.
        p. cm.

        ISBN 0-9661826-4-2 (hardcover)

1. Vertigo--Popular works. 2. Dizziness--Popular
works. I. Poe, Dennis.

        RB150.V4C66 2005

        616.8'41--dc22

                                                2005001418

Copyright 2005 by Auricle Ink Publishers

First Printing

ISBN: 0-9661826-4-2

Cover Concept and Design
by Dee Bayro

This book is available at special discounts when ordered in
bulk quantities. Contact the publisher for more information.

Auricle Ink Publishers
PO Box 20607
Sedona AZ 86341
(928) 284-0860
www.hearingproblems.com

DISCLAIMER

This book is intended for use as a <u>supplement</u> to sound medical and/or surgical management. It is not intended as a means for self-diagnosis. If you are working with a physician, audiologist or other healthcare practitioner, this handbook can be very informative about the process you might experience during the exploration of your condition. The editors, authors, contributors and publisher are not responsible for decisions you or your healthcare team make regarding your diagnosis, or lack of diagnosis of your condition, nor choices for treatments you might seek or undergo.

No direction, ideas or suggestions from this book should be made or taken without the expressed consent of your physician, audiologist or healthcare parctitioner who is managing your dizziness or vertigo. You need to work with such a practitioner to gain the most from this book.

Table of Contents

INTRODUCTION

Dennis Poe, MD
Department of Otology and Laryngology
Harvard Medical School, Children's Hospital of Boston
Massachusetts Eye and Ear Infirmary
Boston, Massachusetts

Dr. Poe earned his MD from SUNY Syracuse, his residency in otolaryngology-head and neck surgery at the University of Chicago, and a subspecialty fellowship in neurotology with the Otology Group in Nashville, Tennessee. He is a full-time faculty member in the department of Otology and Laryngology, Harvard Medical School and Children's Hospital of Boston. He is also on staff at the Massachusetts Eye and Ear Infirmary. He has published a number of scientific research articles and patient information writings on medical and surgical treatments for Meniere's disease. He has done pioneering work in minimally invasive surgery of the ear.

Dizziness is one of the most common complaints people report to their physicians. The National Institute of Health has reported that 90 million Americans (42 percent of the population) will present to their doctors with a complaint of dizziness at least once within their lifetime. The cost of medical care for treating patients with balance disorders has been estimated at over one billion dollars per year in the United States alone. Balance disorders become increasingly common as we age. It affects 40 percent of Americans over the age of 75. The number of patients with dizziness increases significantly with age and it represents the leading complaint in patients over the age of 75.

The national ambulatory medical care survey in 1991 found that dizziness or vertigo was among the top 25 most common reasons Americans visited their doctor. Physicians in the U.S. have reported a total of more than five million visits per year for dizziness alone.[1] The good news is that in the majority of cases it can be accurately diagnosed and effectively treated once a comprehensive assessment has been done.

"Doctor, I'm dizzy."
"What do you mean by dizzy?"
*"I don't know. I thought you're supposed to tell me what I
   mean."*

This all-too-common interchange demonstrates a fundamental problem in communication that occurs when people try to discuss *dizziness*. It also illustrates the need for this book. All of us have experienced sensations that we would call dizziness, but everyone has their own impression of what dizziness means. The term can be used loosely for almost any sensation involving our brains, thoughts, consciousness or balance that seems out of the ordinary. It can be quite difficult to convey to another person exactly what you're feeling when you're dizzy.

A recent encounter with one of my patients began with her making circles in the air with her finger and telling me, "I can't explain my dizziness but I feel something in my head, *you know.*" Unfortunately *we can't know* how you feel inside without you describing it in some detail. It is our hope this book will help you to do just that.

The word "dizzy" is defined in the Merriam-Webster Dictionary[2] as: "1: foolish, silly. 2: having a sensation of whirling: GIDDY. 3: causing or caused by giddiness." The definition for "giddy" is: "1: dizzy. 2: causing dizziness. 3: not serious: frivolous, silly." The English language does not offer any help to us in trying to express our sense of dizziness to one another through this word since it is defined in terms of giddiness, and "giddy" is defined in terms of dizziness. Another serious problem is the alternative connotations of foolish, silly and frivolous. These can add a serious stigma that contributes to anxiety, frustration and social isolation experienced by someone who suffers from dizziness.

In order for you to be helped with a dizziness complaint, we medical practitioners need to understand as precisely as possible how you're affected by the problem. Most of the diagnoses for dizziness conditions can be made on your history alone, so accurate communication between you and your physician is a crucial part of the process.

How This Book Can Help You

The principal purpose of this book is to help you or someone you know who suffers from dizziness to be able to better communicate what you feel to your doctor, medical caregivers, and even other non-medical people. The ability to communicate what you feel more accurately will greatly aid medical personnel in arriving at an accurate diagnosis and appropriate treatment. It will also help others understand your condition and remove some of the barriers that occur when someone suffers from an illness that is not felt or seen by another person. There is no means for measuring the quality and severity of symptoms we feel such as pain or dizziness. This book is designed to help you express what types of symptoms you have and understand what information your doctors will be looking for in trying to diagnose and treat your condition. The pattern of dizziness complaints and associations with other symptoms or illnesses are important in arriving at a diagnosis. This book will also provide a great deal of information about what to expect from your doctor and the medical system as you are evaluated for your dizziness problem.

Dizziness can be due to a staggering number of disorders that may include the cardiovascular system, the central nervous system, the vestibular or balance system (including the inner ear) and other systemic problems such as metabolic or hormonal abnormalities. Table 2-1 (on page 37) lists the top possible causes for dizziness (called a differential diagnosis) from a commonly used textbook of internal medicine. The list is not only long, but many of the disorders are frankly scary, such as strokes, brain tumors and multiple sclerosis. Fortunately, the most serious conditions are relatively rare.

Your doctor will try to listen carefully to the symptoms you describe and search for the type of system abnormality that most closely fits your symptoms. Most of the time your diagnosis will be apparent on the basis of your history alone. Subsequent physical examination and testing will be done on the basis of what has been discovered during the history in an effort to confirm or deny the initial impression.

This book will take you through all of the steps of the history, physical exam, and the different types of examinations and balance testing available. It will give you an overview of the rationale for why we order various tests and how the results are helpful. The book will also discuss in some detail the most common balance disorders, those involving the vestibular system which includes the inner ear balance (vestibular) organ, the nerves that connect to the inner ear, and the neural centers (nuclei and connecting nerve axons) in the brain that process balance and coordination information. Medical treatments (and when appropriate surgical alternatives) for these more common conditions will be presented.

Not all vestibular system injuries are repairable and for those that are not, this book will discuss the concept of vestibular compensation for injuries and strategies designed to recover as much function as possible. If you suffer from dizziness, you may already realize the tremendous social and psychological stresses and burdens on you. Some people are often unable to perform their normal routines or may actually be disabled. Such stress may seriously detract from someone's ability to cope chronically with a vestibular problem and managing these stresses optimally can help someone function to their best possible performance.

This book is <u>not intended to be a step-by-step guide to self-diagnosis</u>. It is in no way exhaustive of all of the different conditions that can cause dizziness. We have endeavored to cover the most frequently encountered diagnoses in considerable detail and outlined the diagnostic process. Strategies for treatment of most of these common conditions are presented. We hope that you find the book useful in organizing your own thoughts about your condition and understanding the definitions that will be in the minds of your doctor so that you can best communicate your symptoms and patterns of the illness. This team effort between you and your doctor will greatly facilitate an accurate diagnosis and getting you into appropriate therapy.

In the optimal system, a patient may present with a dizziness complaint to their primary physician and receive adequate evaluation and treatment at that level. If the problem is persistent or requires more sophisticated analysis, the primary doctor should have the ability to make the appropriate referrals. As we do not live in a perfect system, a patient will often present to the primary doctor with a bewildering array of symptoms that initiates an evaluation of nearly every possible organ system in the body. Many times this so called "mega workup" may have been unnecessary if the communication between the patient and physician had been better honed in on a limited differential diagnosis.

At the end of a "mega workup," a patient may feel frustrated with the ongoing problem and no definitive diagnosis. Referrals are then made to additional specialists who in turn obtain "mega workups" and accumulate a number of *negative test* results (that is, no medical pathology) all along the way. Anxiety, frustration and even anger can build as one moves from one specialist to another without getting definitive answers. During this time a patient may start complaining of additional symptoms which were not previously important enough to be "on the radar screen." A patient might offer these in the hope that somebody will pick up on something and shout out, "Eureka!" with the final diagnosis and magic treatment.

Unfortunately these additionally lengthy and bewildering collections of symptoms may serve to cloud and confuse the issue. Under such circumstances, referral to an otologist, neuro-otologist or otoneurologist can help cut through much of the frustrating diagnostic process. These professionals are well-trained in trying to help patients focus in on the important aspects of their illness and cut to some important clues as to their underlying problem.

The diagnostic process requires good communication between you and your doctor. Doctors must do everything they can to try to get inside your head and understand what symptoms you have and how severe they are and to look for various patterns that will be helpful in leading to a diagnosis and treatment. You must also listen carefully to what the doctor is asking for and provide information that is as pertinent as possible. It is the hope that this book will help you organize your thoughts and look for what we identify as important symptoms and patterns so that you can relate your problems as accurately as possible. With both doctor and patient doing their very best to listen to each other and find some common language and definitions, we hope we can help each of you to find the best road for you to help yourself through the dizzying world of the dizzy evaluation.

This book is also designed to help you understand how your doctor has arrived at the recommendation for a particular type of therapy and how it's expected to help you. This kind of information can be extremely beneficial for you to do everything you can to help yourself.

My suggestion for optimizing your personal use of this book is to use it as it was designed—as a "Handbook." This means that the only chapters you may need to read are those that apply to your specific situation. A couple chapters cover rather complex aspects of dizziness and vertigo and as a result it's frankly impossible to oversimplify some of this terminology. If you experience this, don't get stuck on unfamiliar words. There's an extensive glossary in the back for your reference. Use it. By the same token, don't overuse it. That is, don't try to capture every word. Each time a word comes up for its first use in this book, it is *italicized*. This will identify that this word or phrase is in the glossary. So long as you understand the concept, you're miles ahead. After all, we're not going to test you on it.

If you've obtained this book through your medical or audiological practitioner, ask for a recommendation of two or three of the most important chapters that apply to you (mark the first insert page of this book). Then, should you be interested in doing so, you may puruse the table of contents or the index to see if there are additional sections you may want to explore on your own.

We are very pleased to have assembled a wonderful group of experts in the field of dizziness. Reading the invaluable information contained in this book might be likened to the rare opportunity of consulting with the most qualified experts in the field of vestibular disorders. They'll provide candid insights into how they approach different aspects of their specialty and try to help you through their perspectives on problems of dizziness and its management. Listen carefully to their advice which stems from decades of experience, but foremost heed the wisdom of your physician who is managing your problem. We also hope you'll find this book helpful to assist you in forming the right partnership with your doctor in your search for the cause and treatment of dizziness or vertigo. You may be pleasantly surprised by much of what you read and how you may be able to at last take control of your problem.

- Good Luck!

References

1. Vestibular Disorders Association (VEDA) website, www.vestibular.org
2. *The Merriam - Webster Dictionary*, Mish, Ed., Merriam-Webster, Inc., 1997

CHAPTER ONE

Normal Operation
of the Balance System in Daily Activities

Neil T. Shepard, PhD
Department of Special Education and Communication Disorders
University of Nebraska—Lincoln
Lincoln, NE

Dr. Shepard is Professor of Audiology in the Department of Special Education and Communications Disorders, University of Nebraska–Lincoln and a member of the faculty at the Boys Town Research Institute in Omaha. He received his undergraduate and masters training in Electrical and Biomedical Engineering from University of Kentucky and Massachusetts Institute of Technology. He completed his PhD in auditory electrophysiology and clinical audiology from the University of Iowa in 1979. He has specialized in clinical electrophysiology for both the auditory and vestibular systems. Activity over the last 20 years has concentrated on the clinical assessment and rehabilitation of balance disorder patients and clinical research endeavors related to both assessment and rehabilitation.

Overview

The sensation of dizziness, whether that is a spinning of your world, lightheaded feeling, imbalance or a combination of these symptoms constitutes a significant public health problem in the United States and elsewhere. Estimates of the number of persons in the U.S. seeking medical care for dizziness range as high as 7 million per year. Approximately 30 percent of the U.S. population has experienced episodes of dizziness by age 65. There are no indications that the problems of dizziness and imbalance are diminishing, particularly as the population ages. Having an understanding of the daily function of the balance system is important in the comprehension of what causes symptoms of dizziness and imbalance. This knowledge also helps in the understanding of how patients with these complaints are evaluated and treated. This chapter presents information about how the normal balance system is supposed to function. It is intended to support your reading of the remaining chapters that discuss specific disorders of balance and dizziness and techniques for evaluation and management of those conditions.

What is the Balance System?

No single structure makes up or controls balance system function. Rather, the balance system consists of three structures that gather information about how we are moving, oriented to gravity (standing on our feet or our head) and how the world around us is moving. These three input (sensory) structures are:

1. the balance organ portion of the inner ear, called the *vestibular endorgan* (the other portion of the inner ear is involved with hearing);
2. our eyes; and
3. information from the soles of our feet and our joints (especially the ankle, knee, hip and neck) called *proprioception*.

The input information is brought together at a level in the back of the brain in two specific structures called the brainstem and the cerebellum. The input information results in routine responses for eye movement, maintaining upright stance and perceptions about how you are moving.

When considering function of the balance system, it's helpful to look at the major purposes that the system attempts to accomplish. You can view these purposes as three distinct areas:

1. Perceptions of how we are oriented in a gravitational field (standing on our feet or our head), the direction and speed of movement and when a change in the movement occurs.

2. Being able to maintain a clear visual image of the world around us even when our head is moving or the scene we want to watch is moving, or both is happening. An example of this is your ability to read a street sign while moving over a rough road. If this aspect of the system was not working, the sign would appear to be bouncing as long as you were moving. This would be similar to watching the sign in a movie taken with an old video camera mounted on the vehicle.

3. Ability to maintain upright stance and to perform movements ranging from routine walking to complicated movements involved in sports, dance, etc. There are two areas that assist this last purpose:

   • Your ability to automatically respond to an unexpected movement of your body occurs without having to think about the activity. For example, standing at a gathering of persons and having someone accidentally bump you while you are talking to another. You sway forward, put yourself back in place and never stop your conversation.

   • The ability to maintain your body positioned over its base of support (this would be your feet while standing, hands if doing a hand-stand, other parts of your anatomy when sitting, etc.) and make planned movements for purposes of routine daily activities or to learn and perform more difficult tasks involved with sports and dance.

For either of these areas, maintaining upright stance and walking, it's important to realize that a fall is defined as having the body become positioned outside of the base of support and not have that position corrected in a rapid enough manner. Under the condition where you are unexpectedly bumped, this would occur if the push was large and you did not take the corrective action of stepping forward or backward to adjust. In the situation when voluntary movements are being made such as walking, but you catch your toe on an object and are unable to right yourself quickly, your body would then be outside its base of support and a fall would occur.

It is estimated that while you are walking you are within a third to a half a second of a fall at any time. Therefore, if you catch your toe, you do not have long to react before a fall occurs. This has special implications for us as we age since our reaction time becomes slower. It also holds concern for persons who develop conditions causing them not to be able to feel where their feet are positioned.

How We Control Eye Movements and Develop Our Perceptions of Movement

Of the three input portions of the balance system discussed above, the balance organ in your inner ear is the one with the majority of responsibility for controlling your eye movements when your head is in motion. This also provides the information needed to perceive in what direction you are moving, how fast and how that motion is related to the pull of gravity. Therefore, the inner ear portion of the balance system has the primary job of accomplishing, with the brain, the first two purposes of the system outlined above: the ability to know how we are moving when we are changing our direction and speed, and providing clear visual viewing of our world when moving the head.

As a result of these tasks, if one or both of the balance portions of the inner ears are not functioning properly, many patients will complain that their vision is blurred. They will also complain that they feel movement of their body or the environment around them when they know they and their surroundings are actually still. Because of the visual blurring, especially with head movements, patients think there is a problem with their vision and typically have this investigated, only to find that their vision is working normally. The real problem lies with the inner ear not being able to properly control movement of the eyes when the head is moved. Let's look in more detail at how the inner ear accomplishes this task of eye movement control. As you watch an object of interest that is stationary and your head is not in motion, you position your eyes to maintain the clearest image of the object. If you now suddenly turn your head to the right, your eyes are moved to the right with the head. Yet, you want to continue watching the object that was directly in front of your face before the movement occurred. The inner ear senses this movement to the right (an acceleration of the head to the right) and produces a reflex that causes your eyes to go in the opposite direction with equal speed. In that manner, your vision is maintained on the original object even though the head has now turned to the right. This reflex called the *Vestibulo-Ocular Reflex* (abbreviated VOR) is especially useful in the situations of walking or riding in a car when you're trying to watch an object in the distance and during the movement the position of your head is continually changing. At the same time your vision is maintained steady and clear, you have the correct perception that you have just turned to the right. This is also a direct result of having the inner ear sense these changes in motion and send that information to the brain producing the eye movement reflex (VOR) which then allows for the perceptions of changes in movement that have just been made.

There are times however, when we would not want the VOR to work. Take for example you are trying to read a map in a moving car. The car is slowing down, speeding up, going around turns to the left and right and the road is rough so you're doing some bouncing up and down. All of this is occurring at the same time. If during these changes to your head motion the VOR was to produce the compensatory eye movements we described above, you would not be able to read the map. This is because the map is moving in a manner similar to your head. Therefore, you don't need a complete correction for all head movement changes from the car motion. This on and off behavior, or your ability to override (suppress) the VOR, is a property of the brain's control over the information that it is being sent from the vestibular endorgan of the inner ear. This suppression is also a direct result of your having something to watch at the same time.

If you were placed in a dark environment or if you were to close your eyes, in the example of the car above, you would not be able to suppress the eye movement reflex. An example of this is seen in one of the tests sometimes used by those investigating problems of dizziness. The subject is placed in a chair in a completely dark room. The chair is gently spun in a circle to the right and then back to the left. As long as you have nothing to watch your eyes will move to the left as your head is rotated to the right and the reverse happens as your head is rotated to the left, the eyes move in a compensatory manner to the right.

If for example, the movement continues to the right, the eyes clearly cannot continue going to the left. After a short interval of eye movement to the left the eyes suddenly jerk back to the right in the direction of the rotation. Then the eyes resume their movement to the left, jerk back to the right and so forth. If you were to be watching someone's eyes as this was happening, you'd see this slow movement away from the direction of their rotation and then the fast movement in the direction of the rotation. This repeating "jerk" movement of the eyes is called *nystagmus*. (Editor's note: The word comes from a humorous ancient Greek description of politicians in the senate who started to doze off while sitting. Their heads would slowly drop forward toward the chest, then suddenly jerk back upright.) In this case, the presence of nystagmus and the expected result of rotation in the dark are normal. If you now turn on the lights during the rotation and have the subject watch their thumb or any other object that is moving with them, the nystagmus is absent or suppressed. The presence of nystagmus at other times and particularly changes in nystagmus with head positions and movements are used repeatedly during investigations of persons complaining about dizziness. The nystagmus production, normal and abnormal, gives the examiner clues as to how the inner ear and parts of the brain are functioning.

It would be useful for your understanding of how the vestibular endorgan of the inner ear works to look at it in a little more detail. Figure 1-1 shows the inner ear in a cut-a-way picture of the human head. As you can see, the inner ear is housed within a bone on each side of the head. Think of the inner ear as a tube within a tube (see Figure 1-2). You have the bony tubes within which soft tubes are held in place. Around the soft tubes is a fluid (*perilymph*) that is held within the bony tubes. Inside the soft tubes are the specialized hair cells that sense the motions of our head for the balance endorgan portion, and sense sound waves for the hearing portion.

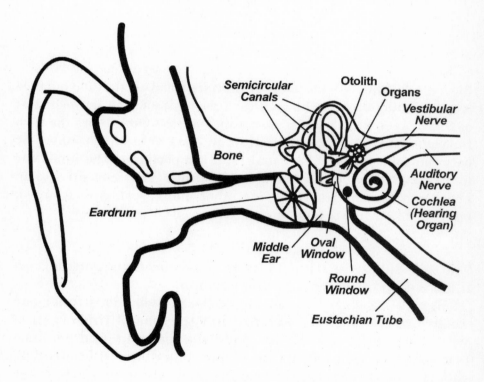

Figure 1-1: Shown is a view of the ear with the skull cut away. It shows the relationship between the outer, middle and inner ear sections. It illustrates the orientation between the inner ear portion for the balance system (vestibular endorgan) and the portion of the inner ear for hearing (cochlea).

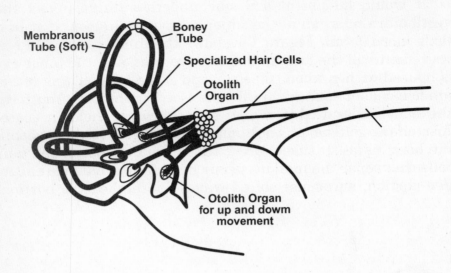

Figure 1-2: This is a close up of the inner ear portion for balance (vestibular endorgan). Shown is the tube inside a tube arrangement of the semi-circular canals. Also note that the Otolith organs (two separate structures) are located in an open area of the inner ear between the semi-circular canals and the portion of the inner ear for hearing. As indicated, one of the Otolith organs is sensitive to up and down movements while the other one responds to forward, backward and side to side movements.

The soft tubes, referred to as the *membranous portion*, are filled with a different fluid (*endolymph*).

Figure 1-2 shows a close-up of the membranous inner ear taken out of the head. Realize that the size of this organ is tiny. The entire inner ear, both the hearing and balance portions, would fit within the surface of a dime. In Figure 1-2, you can see three partial circles coming off the main chamber of the inner ear at different angles. These are called the *semi-circular canals*. As the head is moved in a circular motion, such as making a turn right or left or nodding the head, the fluid within the semi-circular canals moves causing movement of the a jell-like covering (*cupula*) over the hair cells. This results in the movement of the small hairs on these specialized cells. This event occurs in both vestibular organs on the right and left at the same time. The result of the movement of the hairs is a change in the activity on the nerves that connect the inner ear to the brain. It is this change in nerve activity that stimulates the eye movement reflex (VOR) and our perception of how our head movement just changed. The physical arrangement of these six semi-circular canals, three on each side, is such that any movements in a circular manner that you can make are detected by two or more of these canals.

Not all of our movements during our daily routine are in a circular (angular) fashion. How then do we detect a change in our movement forward, backward, to the side, up or down? It's not the semi-circular canals that respond. We have two additional detectors in the vestibular endorgan of the inner ear, one for movements forward, backward, to the sides and one for movements up and down. The positions of these are shown in Figure 1-2 to be in the main chamber of the inner ear and are called the *Otolith organs*. These structures are responsible for detecting linear (forward, backward, sideways, up and down) changes to our movements. These are also the parts of the balance endorgan that respond to positional changes of our head compared to the pull of gravity toward the center of the earth. Therefore, it is the Otolith organs that respond if our head is tilted forward, backward or to the sides and held steady in that position. Like the semi-circular canals, the Otolith organs have specialized hair cells that when the hairs are moved cause a change in the activity of the nerves from these detectors to the brain. However, in the Otolith organs there is a difference in the jell-like substance that covers the hairs from the hair cells. The covering substance contains small crystals imbedded in the jell making it heavy compared to the fluid around the Otolith organs.

Therefore, if the head is tilted forward, the jell-like covering moves because it's pulled by gravity to a new position even though the head is steady. This results in a movement of the hairs from the hair cells and a signal is sent to the brain from both the right and left sides. This signal results in an eye movement reflex that raises the eyes to keep them looking straight ahead and the perception that the head is now tilted down. In this example, since the head is in a stationary position (tilted down), the semi-circular canals do not respond, since the jell over those hairs moves only when the head is moving and doesn't respond to the pull of gravity.

In the next chapter and throughout this book, a condition called *Benign Paroxysmal Positional Vertigo* will be referred to. In this disorder, crystals make their way into the semi-circular canals and for a period of time cause them to be sensitive to gravity when that is not the manner in which they were designed to function. If you ever have the opportunity to travel into outer space, you would find that you continue to detect angular (rotational) movements in the same way as you do on earth. You could also detect movements forward, backward, sideways, up and down in the same manner as you would on earth. However, unless you have your eyes open you would not be able to tell if you were upside down or right side up compared to the space ship interior, since there is no pull of gravity. Therefore, the Otolith organs now have no means of detecting the stationary position of your head.

It's important to realize that the only movements that stimulate the semi-circular canals or the Otolith organs, giving the eye movement reactions and the appropriate perceptions, are those that involve speeding up (acceleration) or slowing down (deceleration). In other words, if you're moving in a circular or linear manner at a fixed speed, not increasing or decreasing your speed, the vestibular endorgan is not being stimulated and you have no VOR. Your perception is that of being still. The best example of this is when you're flying. As you take off or land you perceive the motion because the aircraft is increasing or decreasing its speed. Yet, when the cruising altitude is reached and it's a smooth flight, vision is clear and your eyes are stable in your head as long as you're looking inside the aircraft cabin while not moving your head on your body. Even though the airplane is traveling up to 500 miles per hour you have no perception of motion. The critical factor in this example is that at the cruising altitude the plane is at a fixed speed. You can summarize this concept by saying that the balance organs in the inner ear only react to changes in your speed of movement, or your stationary head position (whether the head is tilted in any direction from straight up and down).

While the balance endorgan of the inner ear is an extremely useful device and provides a wealth of information about your movements, it clearly needs some assistance when you're not changing your speed, yet are moving. What does this tell us about the direction of motion and the fixed speed at which you are moving? Think about driving on a long straight road in a car with automatic cruise control. You set the speed at 60 miles per hour and for miles you have to make no turns. You perceive your direction of movement and your speed correctly, as long as you have your eyes open! If your eyes are closed and it's a smooth ride, this perception is gone. Below we consider additional mechanisms to the inner ear from our visual input that allows us to develop perceptions of movement when the speed of movement is fixed. These visual systems also assist the VOR in keeping our visual world clear.

The additional mechanisms that assist in control of eye movements all function independent of the vestibular endorgan and the VOR. The one that is the most powerful in producing perceptions of movement is the *optokinetic* system. The purpose of this system is to maintain clear visual imaging of the world when the head is motionless or moving at a constant speed. The optokinetic system is activated when objects move repeatedly across your visual field. This happens when your head is motionless and objects are moving, like that of a passing train. The system is also activated when objects are motionless and you're moving at a constant speed, as in the example above—driving on a flat straight road.

Lastly, your head could be in motion at a fixed speed while objects move at a different speed. An example of this would be driving at a fixed speed and having a train moving alongside the car. The system functions by allowing you to watch one of the many passing targets for a brief time and then moving to the next one, and so on. The system also functions when you're watching a large viewing of a moving scene, giving you the sensation that you're in the scene. The perception of motion, from either the passing of repeated objects or the entire moving scene, can be generated with optokinetic stimulation so powerful that the symptoms of motion sickness (nausea and vomiting) can be produced without you actually having to move.

Most people have experienced optokinetic stimulation in their daily routine or in leisure time activities. You're sitting on the inside lane of a four lane road at a stop light waiting for it to change. The car next to you pulls forward to make a right turn. What is your reaction to their movement? Usually, we step on or press harder on the brake. This response is because we perceived, incorrectly, that we are rolling backwards as a result of the optokinetic stimulation from the car pulling forward. If you have the opportunity to watch people on a train platform who are not taking the train which is about to leave, you'll see them involuntarily lean in the direction of the departing train. Like the car example, as the train begins to move, their immediate perception is that they're falling in the opposite direction so they lean to correct the perceived movement.

In both of these examples, your realization of what is correct (your car is not rolling and you are not falling) comes very quickly. At this point if a second car makes a right turn or another train leaves you do not react. The most powerful example of the visual influence that an optokinetic stimulus can have is in the way this stimulus is exploited commercially in amusement park attractions that simulate motion. Whenever you participate in an attraction that makes you feel that you're moving when this is not the case, there's a large-screen projected image for you to watch. The image on the screen is what is moving. If you go through the ride a second time with your eyes closed you realize that there is no movement other than minor tilting motion of the seats to enhance the effect.

Optokinetic stimulation produces a very accurate response as to the direction and speed you are traveling as long as objects that pass in your visual field are within a 5-10 foot distance and are not moving. This is the example presented earlier about driving on a straight highway at a fixed speed. However, consider the situation of the airplane at cruising speed with a smooth flight. As long as you look within the cabin there is no perception of motion. If you gaze out the window on a clear day, you have a perception of the direction being traveled but your perception of the speed is incorrect since the stationary objects forming the reference are some 25,000-35,000 feet away. If you have broken clouds outside the window your perception of the aircraft speed is far more accurate. During the optokinetic stimulation with repeated moving objects across the visual field, an eye movement is produced called *optokinetic nystagmus*. It appears like that caused by the stimulation of the inner portion of the balance system when the person has nothing to watch. As objects move from the observer's right to left, you see a slow eye movement from right to left and then a fast resetting movement of the eyes to capture the next object to be observed. This produces the slow/fast eye movement combination referred to as nystagmus. Just as in the case of nystagmus produced by stimulating the inner ear, the nystagmus produced by optokinetic stimulation can also be used during investigations of a dizzy patient.

A second means for controlling eye movements and assisting in the production of a clear visual scene is a mechanism that permits tracking of a visual target with a smooth continuous movement of the eye with or without head movement. In general, this is how you'd watch a flock of birds fly across the horizon. To illustrate the use of this control system mixed with the use of the VOR try the following. Hold your thumb at a full arm's length in front of your face. Hold your head still and very slowly move your thumb back and forth in a small arc. Slowly begin to increase the speed of your thumb's movement until it becomes blurry. Now hold the thumb still and very slowly begin moving your head back and forth left

21

and right. Slowly increase the speed of your head until again your thumb is blurry.

First, which could you move faster and keep your thumb in clear focus—your head or your thumb? After a couple of trials all agree that the head could be moved more rapidly than the thumb and be able to keep the thumb clearly in focus. Secondly, what mechanisms are being used to keep the thumb in clear focus during the above experiment? While the head is motionless and the thumb goes from no movement up to the point of becoming blurry, you're using a smooth tracking system called the *smooth pursuit system*. At the point where the thumb is no longer clear, the smooth pursuit system is reaching its limits of function and other mechanisms take over to continue to track the thumb, but not in a clear fashion.

From the prior discussion on VOR, while the head is moving at an average speed up to where the thumb becomes blurry, you're using the stimulation of the inner ear (VOR) to keep the thumb clear in your vision. However, at the beginning with the very slow repetitive head movements, your speed is too slow for the inner ear to effectively keep the eyes on the target. It is at these very slow speeds that the smooth pursuit system assists by keeping the target in clear focus. As the head speed increases, the smooth pursuit system drops out and the VOR takes over.

The *saccadic system* of eye movement control is a final mechanism that we need to consider. The primary function of saccadic movements is to rapidly move the eye and position your focus on a target of interest. This is the system that takes over for the smooth pursuit system when it can no longer keep up with the target being followed. In the experiment above with thumb movement, while moving the thumb with the head still, the thumb became blurry as the saccadic system was taking over. Whenever you want to watch an object that does not have a predictable movement, the saccadic system comes into play.

Consider the idea of tracking a flock of birds flying across the horizon. The smooth pursuit system works very well in allowing you to visually follow the flock. But, have you ever tried to watch bats in flight as they move to catch insects? Their flight pattern is anything but smooth and predictable. Therefore, to follow a bat's movements you would use the saccade system. In order to accomplish this type of tracking this system must be fast and very accurate. In fact, second to a sneeze, the saccadic eye movements are the fastest bodily function you have. An object can move from your view directly in front to the side by 30 degrees, you can reposition your eyes on that object with a single movement that approaches a speed of 500 degrees per second and miss the target by less than a quarter of a degree.

The three eye movement control systems we have just discussed are all controlled by areas of the brain and work in a completely independent manner from the inner ear system, yet complimenting the VOR system. Just as the inner ear system is investigated by examining how the VOR is functioning, the study of the optokinetic, smooth pursuit and saccade systems provide a window into how well certain regions of the brain are functioning.

In our daily routine, we clearly do not pick and choose which of the mechanisms of eye movement control and perception we want to use. All of these *oculomotor* control systems are used in harmony as we attempt to visualize targets of interest during daily activities. Take for example a target of interest moving from straight ahead to a far right position. To continue to watch the target, you send signals from the brain to produce a rightward head movement and rightward saccade eye movement at the same time. Since the eye can move significantly faster than the head, the VOR system is turned off allowing the saccade to focus the eye on the target. The head is then moved to point the nose toward the object. To accomplish this and have the target remain in clear focus the eyes must stay fixed on the target during the head movement. A combination of smooth pursuit and the vestibulo-ocular reflex are used so the target is viewed clearly during the head movement. Once the head and eyes are again stationary, the task is that of maintaining gaze on the target.

This is the process used as we survey the visual world throughout the day. The ability to perform these visual tasks quickly and accurately depends on proper function of both the inner ear and specific brain areas. Abnormalities in any of these systems can produce functional disability for any task requiring coordinated movements of the head and eyes, such as driving a rapidly moving car. This activity demands that the driver constantly monitor the visual surroundings and occasionally glance for information from the dashboard. Knowing the complexity of these seemingly simple tasks helps us to understand why patients with chronic inner ear or brain area dysfunction may feel hopelessly insecure about driving, even when they are not experiencing active spells of spinning or lightheadedness.

Maintaining Upright Stance

We've spent a considerable period in discussion of how we perceive movements and how we maintain clear visual images of our moving world. But how do these systems relate to our ability to stand, walk and make complex movements that are learned for dance, sports etc? At the beginning of this chapter, two mechanisms for maintaining balance were introduced. Let's return and consider each of those in more detail and then discuss the roll of the inner ear and vision in the functioning of these mechanisms.

Take a closer look at your ability to automatically respond to an unexpected movement of your body without having to think about the activity. What workings of the balance system give you the capability to perform the following example that was introduced above? You are standing at a gathering of people when someone accidentally bumps you while you're talking. You sway forward, put yourself back in place and never stop your conversation.

There are actually three system characterizations that come into play allowing this event to occur as described. First, the balance system learns to perform rapid, automatic responses, in reaction to a specific single or combination of inputs from our joints, inner ears and vision. We develop a catalog of these responses and use them when the inputs to the system match what has been learned. The learning occurs as we repeatedly attempt to perform a task. Much of this occurs in our early years as we learn to stand and walk and then expand those skills to more difficult situations. In the example above, the working of this automatic response can be seen by looking at which muscles are activated to move you back into position after the bump caused you to sway forward. During a small, easy, unexpected sway forward, the muscles in the back of the legs and then the ones in the lower back contract starting near the foot and moving up the leg into the lower back to pull you into position. There are actually a large number of combinations of muscles that could be used in this task, but virtually all normally functioning people will do the same thing. This event takes place far too rapidly to allow for the person to consciously consider what to do and then activate the appropriate response. In other words, this is an automatic response.

The second feature is your ability to change this automatic response before it is initiated to match the environment in which you are standing. Consider what would happen if you were standing on an uneven surface such as broken concrete where the entire bottom of your foot was unable to be in contact with the ground at the same time. Now you're bumped from behind and you sway forward. The response now is that of muscles of the upper front of the leg and the stomach area set into activity at the same time. The result is your hips are thrown backwards counteracting your sway forward and pushing you into position. This looks more awkward to an observer and requires more work on your part, but is very effective in preventing a fall. The change from one type of movement to another to accomplish the same task is a direct result of the difference in the surface on which you are standing. The surface environment signals a need for a change in the reaction before it is required.

What happens if you're standing on an unfamiliar surface and your sensory inputs misinterpret the situation? Your automatic reaction could make you more unstable. This is where the third consideration comes into play. This third characterization allows the system to be adaptive to new situations that are not typical in the person's repertoire of input/response combinations. For example, a man is walking and steps unknowingly onto a sudden upward tilt of the surface on which he is walking. This type of sudden change of the foot being tilted upward is one of the typical inputs that signal a need to react to a sway forward. This type of reaction would cause the muscles in the back of his leg and lower back to pull him backwards.

However, in this example the man did not sway forward, but simply had his foot tilt in an upward direction without warning. Yet, since the reaction is automatic, this is exactly what happens, causing an increase in a person's loss of balance, not a correction of balance. In a very short interval of time the balance system realizes it has made an error and sends a corrected response to appropriately restore balance before a fall occurs. If this same situation were to occur in a repeated manner the balance system would change its mapping of what should happen when the foot is tilted in an upward direction.

Therefore, this is a learning system that can be modified by repeatedly exposing an individual to new and different standing conditions. Later in this book is a discussion of the use of a treatment option called *vestibular and balance therapy*. It is the modifiable nature of the balance system, not only for standing but also for inner ear and visual motion stimulation of eye movements that is taken advantage of, in part, in the exercises that are done in this therapy treatment approach. It is these three features that allow us to react rapidly and accurately to prevent falls in our daily routines when we experience unplanned body movements.

How do we learn to perform the planned movements that we execute on a daily basis? What gives us the ability to learn highly complex movements involved in sports, dance, leisure activities such as hiking over rough surfaces, mountain climbing etc? It has been suggested that we use several basic reflexes to learn purposeful voluntary movements. One of these is a complement to the inner generated eye movement reflex—the

VOR—discussed earlier. In this case if you're suddenly moved in a sideways direction while standing, you extend the arm and leg in the direction of movement and draw up the arm and leg on the side opposite your movement. This has the result of pushing you back into your normal stance position. The input that causes this event is also from the inner ear, specifically the structures that respond to straight movements, the Otolith organs.

There is another reflex that causes this same response with extended arms and legs on one side and drawing up the others, but it's not related to moving the head. This reflex is stimulated by the position of the head on the body and not related to the pull of gravity. It's called the *tonic neck reflex* and can be seen in babies as an isolated event, but is not easily detected beyond the age of about six months. It works by turning the head to a fixed position looking to the right or the left. The arms and legs on the side to which the head is turned extend and ones on the opposite side contract. The combination of this neck reflex with the rest of our inner ear balance responses produces characteristic postures that can be seen in dance routines, reaching to catch a ball, when running, turning a corner and so on.

One last basic reflex to be considered assists us in maintaining the posture of our head position as our body moves forward, backward, left, right, up or down. This is called the *head righting response*. It effectively helps to maintain a straight line of vision by keeping your head horizontal as your body is moved. Take the example we considered earlier where you suddenly sway forward, either unexpectedly or in a planned movement. If you keep your feet in one place, as your chest moves forward and tilts toward the standing surface, your head goes in the opposite direction so that it stays level with the horizon and helps to maintain a straight line of gaze. You could guess that this occurs because you have something to watch and yet research shows this happens even if the eyes are closed. This head righting response happens even if the body and head are moved slowly. This response is also a property of the inner ear Otolith system and works by keeping the head aligned with the pull of gravity to help with straight gaze. As you watch sporting events or dance routines, look for these body postures described and realize they are learned behaviors resulting from these underlying basic reflexes.

How do the Inner Ear, Vision and Information from our Joints Contribute to Upright Stance?

When walking or standing in a quiet manner, your ankle and knee joints and information from the bottom of the foot assist in your upright stance control and volitional movements. The joint inputs (information) are more often utilized than inner ear and visual inputs for these simple tasks, with the inner ear and vision increasing their influence as the skill level or complexity of the task increases and/or desired speed of movements increase. This is clearly seen by observing the contrast in normal stance and difficulty walking of an individual who is without inner ear inputs in a dark environment. Individuals will widen the separation of their feet as they walk to increase the size of their support surface to make up for the absence of inner ear inputs and vision in this difficult walking situation. However, if these same individuals are asked to stand quietly, a much simpler task, with the feet together and the eyes closed, this can often be done in a normal fashion.

There are, however, individuals who have lost feeling in their feet and at the joints of the ankle and sometimes the knee. In this situation the person sways more than expected when standing still with eyes closed. Since the inner ear information is not as effective as the joint information in maintaining quiet stance, an increased amount of sway results. Yet when walking in a lighted or darkened situation, such an individual can do both in a normal manner.

These same contrasts are true for a person reacting to a sudden unexpected movement in body position. In our example of the person at a party who is bumped from behind, if all systems are working, (inner ear, joint and vision input) they rely primarily on the joint input to initiate the types of muscle activity described above. If joint inputs are reduced because of disease or simply standing on soft surfaces (like thick carpet or grass), the trigger for the reaction must come from the inner ear, in which case it takes longer to start the needed response. In this way one input system can substitute for another in a limited manner.

The visual system, while important, is not critical to upright stance or walking unless one of the other two systems is unavailable or damaged. Yet, as in the train example when discussing optokinetic stimulation, the influence that visual stimuli may have over postural control can be significant. This is especially true if objects equal to or greater than a person's height are within 15-20 feet away. Typically the visual influence occurs in the form of optokinetic stimuli. As we stand or walk through an area of congestion with other people moving about such as in a mall, the optokinetic stimulus effect is continuous. For most people, this effect is suppressed by ignoring the moving objects, using our joint and inner ear inputs for reference as to how we are moving and if needed, looking at objects that are not moving.

However, this situation produces significant symptoms of imbalance for some patients. For these patients, head or eye motion with fixed objects in the visual field can be equally stimulating. The most common example involves the subject walking through the aisle of a store and looking at the objects on the shelves, the "grocery store effect." For many who are sensitive to visual motion stimuli, the symptoms of imbalance and being disoriented by the visual motion can be stronger than those stimulated by head movement.

Changes in our daily environment for standing, walking and making other movements should produce appropriate changes in the coordinated output responses to the three input cues of inner ear, vision and joint information. However, they may also place the inputs into direct conflict with each other. It is suggested that information from vision or joint inputs (that agree with the inner ear information as a reference) is maintained while conflicting information is suppressed. Obviously, some time is required for this process to take place. During this interval, the sensory input conflicts are analyzed and the automatic reaction is modified accordingly.

The example introduced earlier (about what happens when you're stopped at a traffic signal and a car or truck in your side vision begins to creep forward) is a good illustration of the conflict issue. Your reflex is to rapidly apply the brakes in response to a false sensation of backward motion. The optokinetic visual input produced an inaccurate perception of motion, triggering a learned but incorrect automatic response. It is quickly apparent that you're not moving backward and then you release the brake.

If the same event is repeated immediately, the incorrect response will not be produced. Such sensory conflicts are common during daily activities. While most conflicts are produced by visual input, others occur through the joint input pathways. This may occur when standing or walking on an irregular or easily compressible surface (such as gravel, mud, or a soft rug). The normal balance system handles these conflicts with only minor problems. The ability to modify the automatic output responses produced by a particular stimulus in changing environmental situations demonstrates the significant flexibility that is available in the balance system.

How Do You Adjust
If Parts of the Balance System are Damaged?

The inner ear system is the only special sensory system in which loss of function in only one inner ear seriously threatens the well-being of an organism. In humans, injury to specific brain regions (brainstem or cerebellum—areas in the lower back portion of the skull) or inner ear system may result in considerable disability. Fortunately, most disease processes involving the vestibular endorgan are self-limited and spontaneous functional recovery can be expected in an individual who is otherwise healthy. This is due to the remarkable ability of the brain system to recover after inner ear injury, a process known as *vestibular compensation*. Failure to recover from an inner ear insult may be due to ongoing changes in the vestibular end-organ itself or to problems in the brain's ability to drive the vestibular compensation process.

In general, the activity needed in a normal functioning brain to get the compensation process to work is movement of the head and eyes that usually causes symptoms of dizziness. Therefore, in most patients the natural tendency is to not make a movement that causes a symptom. However, the balance system typically needs movement to show the brain what is not working. The brain can then make the compensation adjustments needed to eliminate the symptoms provoked by the movement. The most common reason for the compensation system to fail to be completely effective is restriction in head movement activity on the part of the patient. If the compensation system is not working in spite of the patient's attempts at not restricting movement, then other causes such as those mentioned earlier are investigated.

In summary, the balance system is a remarkable set of mechanisms made up of many components. These work in a very complex and coordinated manner to allow you the ability to move in simple to highly difficult ways. Despite movements of the head and the scene around us, we should be able to maintain clear visual imaging at the same time. The complexity of the system in its normal operation is one of the reasons that the same symptoms expressed by a patient may have many different causes. The remainder of this text explains the processes and the information that is gathered to sort out what can be a very large and complex puzzle in order to arrive at an accurate diagnosis and determine the appropriate management strategies for patients reporting symptoms related to balance and dizziness.

Suggested Further Readings

For the reader interested in more technical details of the normal functioning of the balance system, the introductory chapters in the following textbooks offer the opportunity to significantly expand on the information provided in this chapter.

1. Goebel JA, ed. Practical management of the dizzy patient. Philadelphia: Lippincott Williams & Wilkins, 2000.

2. Shepard NT & Solomon D. Practical Issues in the Management of the Dizzy and Balance Disorder Patient. Otolaryngologic Clinics of North America June 2000; 33(3).

3. Herdman, SJ. Vestibular Rehabilitation. 2nd ed. F.A. Davis Co, 1999.

4. Shepard, N. & Telian SA. Practical Management of the Balance Disorder Patient. Singular Publishing Group, Inc., 1996.

5. Jacobson, Newman, & Kartush. Handbook of Balance Function Testing. Mosby Year Book, Inc., 1993, (Now published by Singular Publishing Group, 1997).

6. Baloh & Honrubia. Clincial Neurophysiology of the Vestibular System, Edition 2. FA Davis Company, 1990.

7. Bronstein, Brandt & Woolacott. Clinical Disorders of Balance and Gait. Oxford University Press & Arnold, 1996.

CHAPTER TWO

Diagnosing Dizziness and Vertigo–History

Dennis Poe, MD
Department of Otology and Laryngology
Harvard Medical School, Children's Hospital of Boston
Massachusetts Eye and Ear Infirmary
Boston, Massachusetts

Dr. Poe earned his MD from SUNY Syracuse, his residency in otolaryngology-head and neck surgery at the University of Chicago, and a subspecialty fellowship in neurotology with the Otology Group in Nashville, Tennessee. He is a full-time faculty member in the department of Otology and Laryngology, Harvard Medical School and Children's Hospital of Boston. He is also on staff at the Massachusetts Eye and Ear Infirmary. He has published a number of scientific research articles and patient information writings on medical and surgical treatments for Meniere's disease. He has done pioneering work in minimally invasive surgery of the ear.

This chapter is divided into two sections: first definitions, then how to think about the history of your vertigo problem. The definition of *dizziness* itself is quite troublesome. We in the medical field tend to think of the word *dizzy* as being a general catch-all term for not feeling whole, alert, well and in balance. The term is far too broad to be useful. We prefer to try to use other words with more limited definitions to start narrowing down what you may be feeling when you're complaining of dizziness. Many patients will admit that they feel "lightheaded" or "heavy-headed." Although still quite vague, these terms convey some sense that a patient is not feeling entirely alert or in control of their sense of well-being. We sense that if these symptoms worsened, it might induce fatigue, drowsiness or somehow alter your sense of awareness of surroundings. More severe lightheaded or fatigue symptoms might lead you to feel *faint*—a sensation that you may be close to *blacking-out* (that is, losing consciousness entirely).

A *near faint* is often experienced when you stand up too quickly and feel a "rush" in your head while your heart and blood vessels are rapidly responding to your head's change in elevation and trying to get the blood up into your head as quickly as possible. This type of lightheadedness is quickly relieved usually by simply putting your head back down or sitting down temporarily. If you don't put your head down and the symptoms continue to worsen, you could be in danger of fainting or losing consciousness.

Some people prefer the term *woozy*. This seems to have a stronger sense of losing control and touch with your surroundings than being just lightheaded or heavy-headed. It can imply a feeling of intoxication in that your perception of things is not keeping pace with the real world. You have to work hard at trying to maintain awareness of everything going on around you.

When we talk about vestibular system problems, symptoms can generally be broken down into vertigo, disequilibrium, or imbalance. *Vertigo*, which comes from the Latin verb "to turn," is a technically precise term defined as a hallucination of motion when, in fact, motion is not occurring. This could mean that you feel you're spinning around or moving in some way when in fact you know that you're not. It could also mean that you see things move when you know that they're not moving or you're seeing or feeling motion differently from what you know is actually occurring.

The most common type of vertigo is a *spinning* or *whirling* sensation as noted in the dictionary definition above. This spinning is most commonly in the horizontal plane (that is, level with the ground), but sometimes people will feel rotation in a vertical plane or from front to back. Vertigo can also mean rocking motion such as commonly experienced when one disembarks from a boat. When you close your eyes after riding on a rolling sea you can often feel as though you're still aboard the ship for hours or days afterwards. Someone with a vertigo condition may be driving a car and stop at a traffic light and yet feel the vehicle is still in motion when he or she knows it isn't. When you fall asleep and suddenly feel as though you're falling, this can be a normal occurrence, but still defined within the term of vertigo. Vertigo is not actually a fear of heights or that sense of ill feeling in the pit of your stomach when you peer over the edge of an unprotected height as we saw in the movie "Vertigo" by Alfred Hitchcock.

All of us have experienced vertigo by spinning ourselves around or by amusement park rides that spin us. When the motion stops, we still feel the rotation continuing. If the rotation is overly stimulating, you may develop a queasy stomach (nausea) and in the most extreme cases, lose your lunch. For patients with vertigo spells, remember that a lot of people go to Orlando, Florida every year to enjoy the sensation that you can get for free at home. The tourists are more fortunate in that they can choose the time and place of their vertigo!

Disequilibrium or *imbalance* are similar terms. They refer to a sense that your balance or equilibrium is not functioning properly. You do not have to experience a hallucination of motion. You may find that you're having trouble simply walking and that you need to touch surrounding walls for reassurance. Some people feel they are constantly drifting to the right or left of the centerline of a corridor as they walk or bump into things excessively. Turning the head in one direction or another or even looking upwards or lying down may produce a sense of losing stability without actually provoking a sensation of motion. Some people have a sense of dysequilibrium at all times while others experience it only when they're moving in some way.

Feeling faint, as though you may black out (lose consciousness) is called pre-syncope. A complete fainting spell in which you lose consciousness or black out is called *syncope* (pronounced sin'-ka-pee). Most vestibular conditions or balance disorders will not actually cause someone to lose consciousness. When this occurs it strongly implies there may be a problem with your cardiovascular system or neurological system. It's therefore quite important to differentiate between feeling truly faint and only lightheaded and not about to lose consciousness.

There can be other changes in your mental status causing various degrees of fatigue, confusion, difficulties with memory or arithmetic and other cognitive difficulties. These can be isolated problems or they can actually be induced by dizziness from other causes. Individuals with a vestibular disorder must expend tremendous amounts of energy every day just to help maintain balance and are likely to have increased mental fatigue with cognitive side effects. What results is little energy left over for short-term memory and mental arithmetic. Few people are in their best frame of mind to solve complicated mathematical problems at bedtime. I've reassured countless patients with these complaints that they were not losing their minds or developing Alzheimer's disease but only struggling with limited energy supplies.

Diagnostic Dilemmas of Dizziness

Nonspecific dizziness and lightheadedness can be due to a tremendous variety of disorders. In general, conditions causing true vertigo or disequilibrium will be caused by a disturbance in the vestibular system. The other more generic causes of dizziness and lightheadedness without disequilibrium or vertigo imply other types of problems. A lack of blood supply to the brain is a very common cause of lightheadedness. It can be induced in healthy and unhealthy individuals just by standing up too quickly. Hardening of the arteries to the brain (atherosclerosis) can provoke this type of lightheadedness. It may involve the small blood vessels in the brain or more significant blockage or narrowing (stenosis) of the carotid or vertebral arteries that provide the principle blood supply to the brain. Any type of cardiac condition that reduces blood flow to the brain can induce such symptoms. Even athletes whose pulse runs in the 40s, compared to a normal adult pulse of about 80, might provoke this type of lightheadedness if they jump up too fast and it takes nearly two seconds before the next heartbeat.

Disorders that can cause dizziness and vertigo are listed in Table 2-1. Dizziness might involve the cardiovascular system, the central nervous system, the vestibular system (balance

Table 2-1: Causes of Dysequilibrium and Vertigo[1]

Inner Ear or Nerve Causes (Peripheral)

Vestibular injury (vestibulopathy)
Labyrinthitis
Vestibular neuritis
Acute or recurrent vestibulopathy
Benign positional vertigo
Ménière's Disease
Perilymphatic fistula
Vestibular toxicity from drugs
Labyrinthine or vestibular nerve disease
- Trauma
- Cancer
- Benign tumor
- Infection
- Connective tissue disorder
- Autoimmune disorder
- Otosclerosis
- Middle ear infection

Central Nervous System Causes (Central)

Brain stem decreased blood supply (ischemia)
Cervical vertigo
Brainstem stroke
Benign tumors adjacent to the brain stem (cerebellopontine angle)
Cancer
Loss of nerve electrical insulation (Demyelinating disease, *multiple sclerosis*)
Cranial nerve injuries or degeneration (neuropathy)
Seizure disorders (epilepsy)
Hereditary familial ataxia
- Spinocerebellar degeneration
- Friedreich's ataxia
- Olivoponto-cerebellar atrophy
Other central causes
- Brainstem tumors
- Cerebellar degeneration
- Inflammatory paraneoplastic syndromes

centers in the brain, balance nerves and inner ear), metabolic problems, hormonal problems and other systemic disorders or major illnesses that can have a weakening effect on the entire body and brain. Vertigo and disequilibrium are symptoms most commonly associated with neurological (central nervous system) problems or vestibular system problems. Lightheadedness without vertigo or dysequilibrium would be more likely caused by abnormalities in the other systems and most commonly with some alteration in blood flow or nourishment to the brain.

Lightheadedness is one of the most common descriptions used for someone's dizziness. One of the most common causes for this is lack of blood flow to the brain which will cause alterations in the level of consciousness or thought processes. This type of lightheadedness is especially common in the elderly who have a considerable amount of hardening of the arteries and complain a great deal about dizziness when they stand up and walk.

Dehydration could also result in low blood pressure and lightheadedness. The brain has extremely high metabolic activity that may be affected by things such as low blood glucose levels that occur with hunger, diabetes, and hypoglycemia.

Conditions that affect the central nervous system are capable of causing either general lightheadedness symptoms or specific vertigo or disequilibrium depending on what part of the brain is affected. The brain is divided into various sections:

1. *the cerebrum* is the location of higher levels of thinking, sensation and voluntary movement centers;
2. *the cerebellum* controls motor or muscle activities as well as coordination; and
3. *the brainstem* provides much of the unconscious functions of our brain such as regulating heartbeat, breathing rate, blood pressure, and other autonomic functions.

There are vestibular centers or nuclei in both the brainstem and cerebellum. A neurological condition such as a

stroke, seizures, *migraine, multiple sclerosis,* tumor, or infection (to name a few conditions), or even a simple lack of blood
flow to one of the balance centers in the brain can cause true
vertigo and disequilibrium. Problems affecting the non-
vestibular areas of the brain may be expected to only cause
general lightheaded symptoms. Elderly persons when they
stand up may have a sudden reduction in blood pressure to
the brain because of hardening of the arteries. Their
weakened heart takes longer to respond than a young person's
in compensating and restoring the normal blood pressure to
the brain. The lack of blood flow to the brain may cause some
non-specific lightheadedness. If the problem is not quickly
corrected the lack of flow to the balance nuclei of the brain
may actually induce the sense of true vertigo or disequilibrium, even to the point of causing a fall. We can begin to see
how symptoms of lightheadedness and true vertigo or
disequilibrium can start to overlap with each other, even
when a single system is affected by the simple movement of
standing up.

The vestibular system includes the brain centers or nuclei
that control our balance, the inner ear organ or vestibular
organ, which is the special sensory organ that we use to
perceive balance and movements, and the nerves that carry
signals from the balance organ into the brain. A disorder with
any of these three parts can produce vertigo and/or disequilibrium. The symptoms will have some characteristics of being
affected by motion.

There are different components of the inner ear itself that
can cause different types of balance symptoms. The inner ear
comprises various sections (see Figure 5-1 in Chapter 3 on
page 116 or Figure 7-1 in Chapter 7 on page 170):

- *three semicircular canals* sense rotational
  movements in the three dimensional planes;
- *the utricle* senses motion in a forward and
  backward direction; and
- *the sacculus* senses motion up and down.

A disorder of any of these sensory nerve endings within the inner ear can produce very specific vertigo in the same orientation as the affected part of the balance organ. Some conditions produce symptoms only when you move your head in a certain right or left direction or with a certain type of rotation that might stimulate one or more of these specific nerve endings. Your doctor may need to spend some time inquiring specifically what types of movements cause your problems.

Disorders of the inner ear follow the general engineering axiom accredited to Murphy's Law: "Anything that can go wrong will go wrong." The nerve endings within the inner ear can be affected by degeneration due to aging or degeneration caused by toxic effects of medications or toxins in the environment. Nerve degeneration can occur for familial or genetic reasons faster in some people than others. Injuries of any sort, trauma to the head, viral or bacterial infections, or inflammatory conditions can contribute to damage to these nerve endings in the semicircular canals. The nerve endings or *crista* are connected by small hair-like projections that reach into a gelatinous mass, the *cupula*, that sways in a column of fluid within the inner ear. The fluids move when we move and we perceive our balance through them. The utricle and sacculus additionally contain small calcium crystals at the top of a broad sensory organ called the *macula*. Deterioration of these crystals or detachment of them resulting in them becoming trapped on the side of the crista or sliding around freely within the inner ear can create specific types of vertigo with certain head positions and movements, called positional vertigo.

There are two chambers of fluids within the inner ear. The innermost chamber is called the *endolymph* and bathes the nerve endings themselves. They are completely surrounded by an outer chamber of fluids called *perilymph*. These two fluids must have strict maintenance of different salt balances and their pressures must be tightly regulated for proper balance functioning. A disturbance in the salt balances or in pressure can lead to profound vertigo. An excess in fluid pressure is called *hydrops* and is thought to be the underlying disorder in *Ménière's disease*, a condition in which there is intermittent severe vertigo spells, hearing loss in the affected ear, ringing noises in the ear (tinnitus), and a sense of fullness or pressure in the ear thought to be related to the elevated endolymph pressure or hydrops. Inflammation of the nerve endings and inner ear (*labyrinthitis*) is thought to be caused most commonly by a virus, but also sometimes by bacterial infections. It can also be induced by inflammatory toxins from nearby middle ear infections. Inflammation of the balance or vestibular nerves themselves can cause vestibular *neuritis* (also called neuronitis).

Some disorders may directly affect the vestibular nuclei, such as migraines or atherosclerosis and can cause nearly identical symptoms as inner ear conditions. Although migraines are commonly associated with headaches, they actually are blood vessel spasms that temporarily reduce the blood supply to a certain portion of the brain and may cause visual disturbances, headaches, or vertigo. Low blood flow may occur in the vestibular nuclei due to hardening of the arteries. We can see that there can be any number of problems that can develop within the vestibular system that may cause multiple types of vertigo, dysequilibrium and/or lightheadedness. You can begin to appreciate the difficulty in trying to unravel where the exact problem may be occurring given that many of these symptoms overlap.

The Diagnostic Evaluation

When you present to the doctor's office with a complaint of dizziness, the doctor will immediately start taking a history of your complaints. We try to understand your symptoms from your descriptions and fit them into the definitions that we understand so that we can start trying to pin down whether the complaint is lightheadedness, disequilibrium, or vertigo, or some combination of these. We immediately begin trying to decide which system in your body may be contributing to the dizziness complaint. The history is the single most important aspect of the evaluation and serves to either hone in on a specific diagnosis or at least narrow down the range of possibilities. After obtaining thorough history we will move on to performing a physical examination. A physical exam will usually be tailored to the areas of concern raised by the history.

A specialist will generally perform a thorough evaluation of the systems that are encompassed in their own field and often may refer you to another specialist if your history or physical findings have raised issues that would be more appropriately examined by a different expert. By the end of the physical examination your doctor should have a reasonable idea of the type of problem you may have. He may have arrived at a specific single diagnosis or have limited the possibilities to a few diagnoses that we call a differential diagnosis. He may then opt to obtain some tests.

Testing is usually done with two purposes in mind. It may be to confirm a suspected diagnosis or to eliminate other less likely diagnoses so that we can feel more confident about our initial impression. A third reason for testing which is much less common would be in the event that we don't have a clue what the diagnosis may be and we are starting to search for possible answers. Even under these circumstances your doctor should have some type of reasonable differential diagnosis in mind.

Suspicion of a neurological condition could prompt referral to a neurologist or a neurological subspecialist called an *otoneurologist* who primarily deals with balance problems. More advanced neurological testing may be done on physical examination. Special neurological tests can be requested such as MRI (Magnetic Resonance Imaging) or CT scans (computerized tomography, also known as CAT: computed axial tomography). Electroencephalograms (EEG) or auditory brainstem evoked response testing (ABR or BAER) may be indicated. Evaluation by an *otolaryngologist* (ENT—ear nose and throat specialist) or a subspecialist ear surgeon (*neurotologist*) will usually be recommended if the condition is felt to lie within the inner ear.

Vestibular disorders are divided into peripheral and central disorders. Peripheral refers to the inner ear itself and central disorders refer to the vestibular nerve and vestibular nuclei within the brain. Since these are often indistinguishable by their symptoms, patients with these types of symptoms are often referred to the otolaryngologist to evaluate for a possible vestibular disorder. The otolaryngologist will perform a thorough ear, nose, throat, head and neck and neuro-otologic examination. The neuro-otologic exam is a neurological physical examination tailored to the ear and balance problems as well as to the nerves that exit the brain (called the cranial nerves).

The History

The history you provide to your doctor is the single most important aspect of the entire evaluation for dizziness. Patients often have the sense that technology has become so sophisticated that it will reveal the cause of someone's dizziness if they simply do enough tests or the "right" test. Unfortunately, this is usually not the case and most of us feel that the diagnosis will be arrived at accurately 90 percent of the time on the basis of the history alone. The remainder of this chapter will help you understand what the important issues are that your doctor will be seeking and guide you in reflecting on your experiences so that you may present your problem as best you can. The physical exam and additional testing will be discussed in Chapter 3. These serve to confirm our impression from the history and to be sure that there are no other underlying problems or surprises.

Lightheadedness, Vertigo or Disequilibrium? How to Tell the Difference

As you learned in the Introduction, your doctor will want to start by trying to understand exactly what type of dizziness complaints you have. The initial question is whether or not there is true vertigo, a sensation of either some type of motion occurring when there actually is no motion or an experience of motion that is different from what you see happening around you.

A sense of imbalance or disequilibrium could be described as feeling that your balance is off and that you're not properly oriented in the world around you. There is no sensation of abnormal motion. Instead, you may experience an abnormal reaction to motion, whether it's you moving or something you see moving. You may feel ill at ease with head movements or body movements, or even have some sense of disconnect from the environment, even when you're not moving. All of these varied alterations in your sense of balance or ability to walk and move can come under the heading of dysequilibrium.

Vertigo and disequilibrium are symptoms which tend to be made worse by head or body movements. Head movements can involve going from sitting to standing, turning right or left, looking upward, or any type of movement from one spot to another.

Lightheadedness is a change in how alert and mentally aware you are and how sharp your mental processes are working. Patients with lightheadedness have difficulty with attentiveness, focusing, and concentrating. If lightheadedness becomes worse, patients often complain of beginning to feel faint or woozy. Further worsening could lead to "blacking out" or losing consciousness. All of these symptoms in the spectrum from lightheadedness to loss of consciousness do not involve a problem with balance. It is certainly possible to have complaints of both lightheadedness and vertigo or disequilibrium. Lightheadedness may cause an alteration in your mental awareness and acuity and at the same time you may have a true disturbance in your balance, ability to walk, or start noticing abnormal motion (vertigo). It's very important for you to try and categorize your own symptoms in these terms so you can explain them to your doctor.

Lightheadedness complaints without vertigo or disequilibrium will start sending the doctor looking in the direction of cardiovascular, general medical systemic, or neurological problems. True vertigo and dysequilibrium will immediately focus attention on the vestibular and neurological systems. Your doctor will want to know more about the patterns of your symptoms and what brings them about.

Looking for Patterns

Pattern recognition is one of the most important aspects of your history. The lightheaded patient whose symptoms begins or worsens whenever they sit up or stand up suggests there's a problem with lack of blood flow to the head when moving the head upward. The heart and blood vessels must react to fight gravity when the head is suddenly elevated and if the reaction is too slow, patients will experience lightheadedness. This is a problem especially common in the elderly. All of us have experienced this type of lightheadedness to some degree, noticing a "rush" to the head and darkening of our vision when we stand up too quickly. This is an increasingly significant problem as we age since vascular reflexes are slower and the heart may be weaker. To complicate matters, a lack of blood supply to the vestibular portions of the brain can produce true vertigo or disequilibrium symptoms in addition to general lightheadedness.

Do you experience any changes in your pulse or breathing when you feel dizzy? Do you have palpitations or thumping racing heartbeats at the time of your dizziness? A fast pulse due to a cardiac condition or even anxiety can provoke an alteration in blood flow to the brain and produce dizziness symptoms but not usually true vertigo.

Your doctor will want to know whether your symptoms of vertigo and disequilibrium come on with any type of head movement at all or only specifically when you raise your head to a sitting or standing position. If there's a clear consistent pattern that the symptoms only occur when sitting or standing up and they're relieved when sitting back down or lying down, this is a strong indication that your cardiovascular system is not fighting gravity quickly enough or adequately with position changes. An assessment of your heart, blood pressure and a thorough cardiovascular system evaluation will be warranted.

If your vertigo and disequilibrium occur with head movements turning side to side or looking up and down regardless of whether your head is in a lying, sitting or standing position, then this strongly indicates that gravity is not a factor and the problem may be in the vestibular system itself. It will then be up to your doctor to try to pin down whether the problem is in the vestibular system within the brain or in the inner ear.

Are there any other medical complaints that come to mind that seem to have any bearing on your dizziness symptoms? Do you have any new medical problems or have you had any changes in medications during this time? Ask yourself if your symptoms come at a certain time of day, month, or season. Do you notice any particular time of day when you get dizzy? If so, does it have anything to do with timing of meals? If there is lightheadedness occurring at the times you are hungry it may be that you have low blood sugar (hypoglycemia) at such a time. Is your imbalance worse on awakening or in the evening? Patients with disequilibrium problems fare better when they are generally active and become more symptomatic after a night's rest. They also may have worsening symptoms by the end of the day as they become fatigued and less able to compensate for their chronic dizziness problem that drains their energy throughout the day.

Hormonal changes may cause lightheadedness or disequilibrium symptoms. Some hormones have specific patterns of symptoms at certain times of day. The thyroid gland is important in regulating metabolism. Abnormalities may cause some types of dizziness. For women, there can be hormonal fluctuations at different times of their menstrual cycle and especially at ovulation or during their period (menses). Certain inner ear conditions such as Ménière's disease and migraines are notorious for striking during the few days when a woman is premenstrual.

Do you have any personal history or family history of allergies? Any possibility of dietary allergies? The most commonly suspected food allergies associated with inner ear reactions are in order of most to least common: dairy, eggs, wheat, soy, corn, and yeast. I once had a patient whom I thought had classic Ménière's disease and he couldn't resolve the problem with medical treatments. We had him scheduled for a neuro-surgical procedure called a vestibular nerve section in which we were to cut his vestibular nerve as a definiti' stop his disabling vertigo attacks. During his trea had suspected he might have a food allergy and he tried soɯ food avoidance trials of each of the above foods, one at a time for two weeks each. When he stopped corn, his symptoms resolved and never came back except briefly when he tried corn again as an experiment to be certain of the allergy. I was happy to cancel his operation!

Problems in the late summer or early spring could imply allergies from high pollen counts. Wintertime problems might be associated with dust and mold allergies.

Vertigo or Disequilibrium?

Your vestibular system senses head movements regardless of whether you're lying, sitting or standing. If you're unsure whether the problem mostly occurs with head movements or the acts of standing up and sitting down are the primary problems, then try these maneuvers on your own. Test yourself to see if the symptoms occur when you go from a laying position to a standing position. If this provokes vertigo or disequilibrium, then put your head down between your knees or lie down. If this makes you feel better you are most likely having a problem with circulation to the brain. If getting up makes you dizzy and laying back down makes you equally dizzy, we would be very suspicious of a vestibular system problem. If you could provoke the same vertigo and disequilibrium responses by just lying down or by moving your head while sitting still or lying still, then we would be even more suspicious of vertigo or dysequilibrium.

- Are there times when the tendency to become dizzy is worse than others?
- Does the vertigo or disequilibrium occur in unpredictable episodes or does it occur on some regular basis?
- How often does it occur and when it occurs, how long does it last?

Some people have vertigo spells that last seconds or minutes and others last hours and even days without letting up. Be precise in describing whether you're having true spinning vertigo continuously or whether you have a tendency to develop spinning vertigo every time you move your head or perhaps just a sense of disequilibrium when you move your head.

Associated Symptoms

You also want to look for any associated symptoms that accompany your dizziness.
- Are there any ear symptoms?
- Have you had any change in hearing in one or both ears?
- Is there any noise in your ear that does not belong there such as ringing or other sounds (*tinnitus*)?
- Do you feel anything in your ear at the time of dizziness such as fullness or pressure in the ear?
- Is there pain in the ear at the time of the dizziness?

You may also relate to your doctor that you have symptoms like this at times other than when you're dizzy, but it would be especially important if you notice a pattern of symptoms related to your ear immediately before, during or immediately after episodes of dizziness. This, of course, could suggest that there's a specific ear problem related to the dizziness.

Are there any visual changes that occur with the dizziness? Many patients with significant vertigo notice that their vision will blur while things are moving. They have difficulty focusing, reading, looking at objects in motion or even with motion on a computer or television screen. Are there any visual hallucinations? Patients with classic migraines may notice various types of lights, bright spots, dark spots or blotches, tunnel vision, wavy or moving lines or shapes, sparkles, fireworks, fire flies, or a number of other visual disturbances. If you notice these types of visual hallucinations, do they occur before, during or after your episodes of dizziness? These types of hallucinations are quite common with migraines but can also be associated with other types of neurological conditions.

How Bad is It?

Be prepared to describe how the vertigo affects you.

- Are you lightheaded all of the time, only sometimes when you stand up or every time you stand up?
- Do the symptoms come and go (intermittent)?
- If you have dysequilibrium, is it intermittent or all of the time (chronic)?
- If you have true vertigo, does it occur every time you move your head or just intermittently.
- Does the vertigo occur only with certain head movements?
- Can you have vertigo which occurs all by itself (spontaneously) without any head movement occurring at all? Spontaneous onset of vertigo is truly disturbing because of the unpredictability creates tremendous stress and anxiety over when and where the next episode may occur.
- Can stress itself provoke a vertigo spell? This is common with Ménière's disease and migraines.

Patients will often tell me that they have vertigo that comes on all by itself but when I really probe them with questions, it turns out that head movements are actually causing the vertigo. They simply hadn't previously made the association between simple head movements and their vertigo, but it's an important distinction. Give a lot of careful thought as to whether dizzy spells can occur while you're sitting or lying still, not moving at all or whether the dizziness comes on with movements of the head or eye, or perhaps just by watching objects or television pictures in motion.

Vertigo that is provoked by head motion or seeing things in motion has very different causes from vertigo that can occur all by itself without any head or eye stimulation. Vertigo limited to head movements implies some type of position-induced vertigo, also called *positional vertigo*. It is most commonly caused by a weakness or injury to the vestibular system, especially within the inner ear. Your body will try to compensate for the weakness as best as possible but incomplete compensation will result in you noticing a problem with your equilibrium when you move your head through certain positions or just too quickly. A special type of positional vertigo called *Benign Paroxysmal Positional Vertigo* (BPPV or BPV for short) is due to malfunction of a single balance canal and will be discussed in detail in Chapter 6.

As opposed to vertigo provoked by head movements or seeing things in motion, some people have vertigo that can occur all by itself. This type of vertigo out of the clear blue without any provocation is called *spontaneous vertigo*. The most common types of spontaneous vertigo are *labyrinthitis* and *vestibular neuritis* (also called *neuronitis*). This is a relatively common condition thought to be due to viral inflammation or infection of the vestibular inner ear organ (the labyrinth) or the vestibular nerve itself that connects the vestibular organ to the brainstem. There may be accompanying viral or flu-like symptoms or no other symptoms besides the vertigo. Severe vertigo may be associated with nausea, vomiting or even diarrhea as a direct side effect of the brain's response to abnormal balance signals and not necessarily due to a virus. Labyrinthitis is usually a short-lived event that subsides after hours, days, or weeks. It usually will not recur. Vestibular neuritis is a controversial topic and it's possible that it may be either a single event or may recur. Spontaneous vertigo that recurs is more commonly due to Ménière's disease or vestibular migraines which will be discussed in detail later in the book. Other more unusual causes of spontaneous vertigo could be stroke, epilepsy, inflammatory conditions, infections or tumors to name a few. Your doctor will investigate these possibilities when it seems indicated.

Unraveling Diagnostic Dilemmas

There is a lot of overlap between types of dizziness and their consequences. They confuse practitioners as well as patients. We have to unravel the details regarding the types of dizziness to get to the bottom of the story. This process sometimes makes us feel like Sherlock Holmes looking for clues to the mystery. For example, dizziness provoked by head movements can be very quickly labeled positional vertigo. Many people will immediately assume that positional vertigo must come from BPPV, a specific semicircular canal disorder often treated with head maneuvers. If the vertigo is in fact due to another cause such as Ménière's disease these head maneuvers will only provoke dizziness that is not helpful in the treatment.

Different Types of Dizziness caused by Spontaneous Vertigo

Positional vertigo or disequilibrium can also be consequences of spontaneous vertigo. Patients with true spontaneous (unprovoked) vertigo that occurs without requiring any provoking head or eye movements often have true spinning vertigo which may last for minutes or hours. During this time there can be strong autonomic nervous system reactions which all of us have experienced if you get too dizzy on a carnival ride or motion sick on a trip. There is characteristically some nausea or even vomiting. You may feel cold and clammy and break into a sweat. You may feel a sensation of being flushed or even hot. Under extreme circumstances, vomiting can become quite severe and there can even be associated diarrhea with loss of bowel control.

Once the acute spinning subsides, there's usually some residual tendency to develop short sensations of vertigo lasting seconds or perhaps a minute or two with any kind of head or eye movement for some time after the attack. It's expected that until you make a full recovery, there will be considerable dysequilibrium or problems with sense of orientation or balance when walking. This type of head movement or position-induced vertigo and disequilibrium can last hours, days, weeks and sometimes months after a vertigo spell. Some people develop chronic head movement induced vertigo and/or disequilibrium indefinitely. You should be very careful to analyze for yourself the difference between vertigo which occurs spontaneously, without any kind of head or eye movement provocation, as opposed to subsequent vertigo or disequilibrium stimulated by head or eye movement. Certainly, while you experience whirling vertigo, any additional head or eye movements will make symptoms feel worse and most patients will feel the need to close their eyes and try to lie down until the acute spinning vertigo subsides.

Headaches causing Vertigo and Vertigo causing Headaches

Do you have any kind of headaches associated with your vertigo spells before, during or afterwards? Headaches are commonly associated with vertigo because head movements exacerbate or worsen the sensation of vertigo. Patients may develop an unconscious tension response in the muscles in the side of the neck and in those attaching to the back of the head. The tension is a misguided effort to stabilize your head and thereby limit the movements that may provoke vertigo. These muscle spasms are abnormal and over time can become quite painful, in effect causing a "charley horse" in these muscles. You can examine yourself to see if your neck pain or headaches may be due to this problem. Massage and press deeply with one or two finger tips into the muscles running up and down the back of the neck or back of the head and explore whether you find that the muscles have some unusual tender or sore spots. Press and move your head and neck to see if certain positions exacerbate the pain. If the cause of vertigo is from the vestibular system in the inner ear or brain on one side, it will usually provoke muscle spasms and pain on the same side of your head or neck. You will want to pay attention to whether there's characteristic pain on one side of the head and neck for this reason.

Additionally, muscle tension headaches can result simply from the stress of going through a vertigo attack. Especially susceptible are the temporalis muscles which are large fan-shaped muscles on the sides of your temples used for chewing. We often clench our teeth when we're under stress or anxious. This type of chronic muscle tension headache can also be associated with vertigo.

Headaches not associated with muscle spasms or tenderness might be due to migraines. Migraines are caused by a blood vessel spasm that reduces the blood supply to a part of the brain. That area of the brain may begin to complain and produce symptoms such as visual problems or other sensations, depending on where the brain is affected. If the vestibular system is affected, it may provoke vertigo attacks that look just like a vertigo attack originating from the inner ear. Recall that the inner ear is outside the central nervous system and is referred to as the *peripheral vestibular system*. A migraine originating within the brain or central nervous system would be called a *central vestibular disorder*. Any personal history of migraines or migraines in your family will be important to bring up with your doctor. You will certainly want to pay attention to whether you have any migraine type symptoms and headaches before, during or after your vertigo spells.

Do you have any other neurological symptoms such as unusual smells, tastes, numbness, tingling or weakness anywhere in your head, face or in the rest of your body? Do you get any of these unusual neurological symptoms before, during or after your dizzy spells?

Conclusions

If you fail to notice any patterns in your dizziness complaints, we often suggest keeping a journal when you become dizzy.

- Were you doing any unusual activities?
- Were you unusually hungry?
- What was the duration of the spell?
- How severe was it?
- What associated symptoms did you have, if any?

You'll also be asked to provide details about your past or current medical or surgical conditions, all of your medications, known allergies, use of alcohol and tobacco and about any other ongoing symptoms (review of systems) that may not seem to have anything to do with your condition. This comprehensive information will be reviewed to see if it sheds any light on the origin of your dizziness complaint.

When you have provided your doctor with a good complete history, they should be already clued in on one or a few likely diagnoses. The next step will be to examine you with this differential diagnosis in mind.

References

1. Anderoli TE, Carpenter CCJ, Bennett JC, Plum F. *Cecil Essentials of Medicine*, 4th Ed., Philidelphia: W B Saunders Co., 1997, p. 835.

CHAPTER THREE

Diagnosing Dizziness and Vertigo: The Physical Exam and Balance Testing

Steven A. Telian, M.D.
Professor of Neurotology, Director of the Division of Otology-Neurotology
University of Michigan

Dr. Telian is the John L. Kemink Professor of Neurotology and the director of the Division of Otology-Neurotology at the University of Michigan. He has written extensively in the field of vestibular disorders, including a textbook and 50 articles or book chapters devoted to this topic among his professional publications. As medical director of the Vestibular Disorders Program at the University of Michigan, he founded the Vestibular Testing Center with Dr. Neil Shepard. This became a model vestibular program that contributed to the training of many professionals interested in the evaluation and rehabilitation of patients with vestibular disorders.

Your doctor should have a good idea of the probable diagnosis before even proceeding on to the next steps of examination and testing. Sometimes, your doctor can even make the correct diagnosis without any testing. Since almost all causes of dizziness share some common symptoms, it is the nature and pattern of those symptoms at onset and then how they develop over time that provides the key to correct diagnosis and treatment. So, please be very careful to organize your experiences in your own mind and as previously emphasized, pay careful attention to answer the doctor's specific questions when giving your medical history. Once your doctor has completed the history, he or she will decide what parts of the balance system need to be examined and what tests will be obtained, if any. My goal in this chapter is to help you understand and anticipate what will happen to you during this phase of the evaluation.

The Physical Examination for Dizziness

After a careful medical history, you should receive an examination from an otologist or *neurotologist* (an ear surgeon who has taken additional training in neurology, neurosurgery and skull-base surgery to treat advanced problems involving the ear, inner ear and the region around the ear and the temporal bone). This will include both an examination of the ears, nose and throat as well as a screening neurologic examination related to the balance system. The entire exam portion may be conducted efficiently in about ten minutes, particularly if there are few abnormalities noted.

Examination of the Ears, Nose and Throat

In most cases of dizziness, the ear examination will be completely normal. Even if the ear is the cause of your symptoms, you should recognize that it's usually the inner ear that is malfunctioning. The doctor is only able to see the outer ear, ear canal, eardrum and some parts of the middle ear. However, abnormalities discovered in the middle ear may be very important. Since the eardrum is not transparent (like plastic wrap) but translucent (more like wax paper), it is often difficult to assess what's going on behind it in the middle ear. Using a hand-held *otoscope* (magnified ear light) to examine the ear may be suitable if the ear is healthy, but abnormal ears are best examined under higher magnification and brighter light using a binocular microscope. This provides the doctor with better visibility and depth perception to evaluate the problem. If there is drainage from the ear, the doctor may use the improved vision provided by the microscope to safely suction and cleanse the ear, both for proper diagnosis and to prepare the ear for treatment. If a tumor, chronic infection or enlarging skin cyst (cholesteatoma) are noted, the doctor may order other tests and/or provide treatment of the condition to see if that is the cause of your dizziness.

Assessment of hearing function is quite important in the evaluation of dizziness. The hearing organ (cochlea) is structurally linked to the balance organ. Beyond this, they share a common blood supply as well as sharing inner ear fluids that must be in perfect balance for the ear to function properly. Likewise, the balance and hearing nerves travel side by side through the same canal in the skull on their way to the brain. In fact, they become almost intertwined at the point when the nerves enter the brain. The doctor will make some effort to assess hearing ability, probably at least with tuning forks. A formal hearing test (*audiogram*) or other special tests of hearing function may be required. If an abnormality of hearing is detected in one ear, it's very likely that the same ear is the one causing the dizziness. Sometimes hearing loss is the only evidence that there is an inner ear problem to blame and this finding may allow your doctor to provide curative treatment. This is so important that I require all my patients with dizziness to undergo a hearing test, even if they don't believe they have a hearing problem.

If the appearance of the ear is normal, but the medical history suggests a possible injury to the tiny membranes that retain the inner ear fluids, the doctor may be suspicious of a perilymphatic fistula. Perilymph is the fluid contained in the outer chamber of the inner ear and surrounds the inner chamber that contains endolymph. A fistula is a leakage of the perilymph fluid from the inner ear into the air-filled middle ear. The most common site for the perilymphatic fistula is through the inner ear's round window membrane, which is a thin membrane separating the cochlea from the middle ear.

If the doctor suspects a *perilymphatic fistula*, he will perform what is called a "fistula test." This test involves sealing the ear canal, then gently increasing and decreasing the pressure on the eardrum. These pressure changes produce a similar change in the middle ear pressure. In such cases, the pressure change in the middle ear will irritate your inner ear, provoking dizziness. The doctor will ask you if you experience dizziness with positive pressure, negative pressure or both. There may be another member of the medical staff in the room to observe your eyes during the fistula test, since inner ear disturbances are usually reflected in predictable but abnormal movements of the eyes.

A positive fistula test in one ear may mean that one is present or simply an abnormal sensitivity to pressure changes in the inner ear for some other reason. A negative test does not prove that a fistula is absent since some of them may be intermittent. However, I would advise you to be slow to accept the diagnosis of perilymph fistula in the absence of a confirmatory test, especially if you've never had ear surgery or an injury to your ear. If there is a cholesteatoma visible in the ear, it may be causing dizziness by eroding the protective layer of thick bone that normally encases the inner ear. In this case, the fistula test confirms the exposure of the inner ear to external pressure changes, and a CAT scan is needed to evaluate the depth and location of the erosion into the inner ear.

Although the nose and throat examination is also usually normal, the doctor will do a fairly comprehensive evaluation looking especially for evidence of serious conditions and/or nerve damage in the nerves supplying the face, throat, larynx (voice box) and tongue. These are called the cranial nerves and they exit from the base of the skull to provide nerve input to important functions in the head and neck. If this type of problem is suspected due to symptoms described in the medical history or obvious abnormalities in your voice, this exam is all the more important. If your doctor is unable to see adequately into your throat with a mirror, an examination may be performed using a narrow flexible telescope that is passed through the nose into the throat. This sounds scary but is actually quite safe and not particularly difficult or painful. While the doctor is viewing the larynx you'll be asked to make a singing sound in order to assess the motion of the vocal cords.

The Screening Neurologic Exam

One reason it takes more time and effort to examine someone for dizziness is the fact that the general ear, nose and throat examination rarely provides an answer to the problem. Thus, it's almost always necessary to do portions of the neurologic examination that we all learn in medical school, tailored specifically to look for problems that might contribute to dizziness or imbalance. The exact portions of the exam your doctor will choose to conduct are appropriately tailored to the suspected conditions, based on your medical history. So, if your doctor fails to perform parts of the examination discussed in this section, it may mean that those parts were not pertinent to the nature of your problem or the solution was already found.

I want to briefly review a couple things presented by Dr. Shepard in Chapter 1. Since eye muscles are neurologically linked to the inner ear, examination of eye movements under a variety of conditions will be very important in most cases. The doctor may initially examine your ability to move your eyes normally in all directions. Next, I always look for rhythmic beating of the eyes called nystagmus (which you'll recall is rhythmic oscillation of the eyes). Certain types of nystagmus are typical of particular disorders and this sometimes really helps with the diagnosis.

Nystagmus that beats up and down (vertical nystagmus) suggests that something is wrong in the brain. If the nystagmus is purely side to side in direction (horizontal nystagmus) or if it repeatedly rotates the eyes (torsional nystagmus), we are more suspicious of an inner ear disorder. If your vertigo is fairly recent in onset or if you happen to have an acute spell in the office, you may have what we call *spontaneous nystagmus*. This means that your eyes are moving when you're sitting doing nothing. It allows the doctor to gain some information about where the dizziness may be coming from. If spontaneous nystagmus is not noted, the doctor may try to bring it out by having you gaze to one side, changing your body position or by shaking your head. If this doesn't work, sometimes you'll be asked to wear special goggles called *Frenzel Lenses*. These are like a scuba mask. They have thick "Coke-bottle" lenses that you cannot see through. This eliminates your natural ability to suppress your nystagmus by staring at an object in the room. Not only can the doctor still see your eyes, they are even magnified by the goggles. Thus, even small degrees of nystagmus otherwise undetectable may become obvious to the doctor.

One special type of nystagmus is associated with a condition mentioned in an earlier chapter called Benign Paroxysmal Positional Vertigo (BPPV), a condition that will be mentioned throughout this book but discussed at length in Chapter 6. Any patient who complains of short blasts of dizziness provoked by lying down in bed, rolling over in bed, rapid head motions or chronic feelings of unsteadiness associated at times with these other symptoms, should be tested for this condition. The doctor will lay you down quickly with your head tilted at 45 degrees over the end of the bed and turned to one side. This is called the *Dix-Hallpike maneuver* (or more simply, the *Hallpike maneuver*).

Once the result on one side is noted, then you'll undergo the same test with the other ear down. Dizziness and nystagmus may be produced by this change in position and the nature of the nystagmus tells the doctor which of the semicircular canals within the inner ear is affected. The dizziness should not be any worse than you've already experienced at home and it should not last more than 10-20 seconds. It's very important not to squeeze your eyes shut or change the position of your head when you feel the dizziness coming, since the nystagmus may be brief and may not repeat the second time the doctor does the test. If you're deathly afraid of the dizziness or if you have chronic neck problems, notify your doctor before the Hallpike maneuver is performed. The test may be modified slightly so it's more comfortable for you. If you become dizzy, it should only be for a short time. Surprisingly, most people can repeat the maneuver right away and have much less severe dizziness or none at all. If that is the case, it will also help your doctor make the correct diagnosis. Therefore, try to be understanding if you are asked to do it over and over.

After careful examination for nystagmus under these various conditions, I usually test the cerebellum next. This is the part of the brain responsible for coordination and keeping us properly balanced in response to the inputs coming in from the rest of the nervous system. Testing this part of the brain involves some tasks that may seem a little silly to you, like repeated patting of your hands or perhaps touching your finger to your nose. These things are quite easy for most people, but if you cannot do them properly, a problem in the cerebellum may explain your dizziness or balance problems. Extending this evaluation somewhat, I like to see how well my patients can balance under a variety of increasingly challenging tasks. You may be asked to stand still with your eyes open and then closed (the *Romberg test*). Sometimes this is repeated while standing on foam so that you can't feel the floor very well. This is much more challenging and forces you to rely strongly on your inner ears once your eyes are closed.

Walking tasks allow us to evaluate the coordination of your gait and your general stability. You may even have to walk a straight line in a heel-to-toe fashion, like the drunk driving test. Sometimes my patients even ask me for a doctor's note so the officer knows that I expect them to fail this test even if they haven't been drinking! It's very important to do your best on these tests. Also, you should never pretend to be more unstable than you really are. If the doctor can tell that you are falsely embellishing the severity of your condition, it may never be possible to properly identify and treat whatever legitimate balance problems you have.

One simple and very reliable test I like to use is called the *Fukuda stepping test*. This is a test that involves marching in place with your eyes closed. If you are stable enough to do this test and one inner ear is much weaker than the other, you'll typically rotate gradually toward the weaker ear while you march. If you turn more than 90 degrees toward one side within 50 steps, I consider this a very strong sign pointing to that ear as the weak one. Sometimes if my patient is turning only a little bit, I'll repeat the test after vigorously shaking the head from side to side. This may enhance the abnormal response in people whose brains have already partially adjusted to (or compensated for) the inner ear injury. This test may not be accurate if there's a persistent sound or conversation in the room that the person can use to orient to the direction he or she is facing. The examiner will help to stabilize you or may choose not to continue if you appear to be too unstable to perform this test.

Sometimes, a more extensive neurologic examination is called for when abnormalities are discovered or suspected from the clinical history. For example, sometimes we need to test your muscle strength and/or ability to rise from a chair to see if there's a problem with the muscles contributing to your instability. Formal testing of sensory function in the legs and feet may be needed to determine whether you're getting proper balance information from the lower part of your body up to your brain. If so, the doctor will assess your ability to detect cold temperature changes, positional changes of your foot or toe, and your ability to feel a pinprick or vibration in the feet.

Laboratory Balance Testing

Being referred to a balance testing facility can be a bit frightening, but most people get through the testing quite easily. There's really only one part that will predictably make you dizzy and most labs have learned from experience to do this part last. It's important not to become drowsy during the testing because this may distort the results. If possible, it's best to stop taking all medications that might sedate you at least 48 hours prior to testing. Many patients with dizziness take meclizine (Antivert™) which is mildly sedating. This can be safely stopped for testing. However, some medications cannot be withdrawn suddenly. If you've been consistently taking fairly high doses of an anti-anxiety medication, suddenly stopping this may cause some very unpleasant effects. You should never stop medications used to treat heart or breathing problems, diabetes or other serious medical conditions. Most of these are not sedating and will not interfere with the test results.

When in doubt, consult your physician. If you cannot stop a sedating medication safely, at least skip your morning dose before testing. I would encourage you to plan your schedule so that you can relax around the home and go to bed early the night before testing. Have a light breakfast unless the testing is very early in the day. Do not eat or drink within two hours before the testing.

The rest of this chapter will review various elements of balance testing and what you may experience when undergoing these tests. Remember that only the most sophisticated facilities will have all of these testing options available. However, remember also that it's often possible to arrive at a correct diagnosis based on the office examination alone.

So why do doctors order balance testing at all? Primarily, it's done for patients with longstanding problems and persisting symptoms despite prior treatment attempts. Sometimes an unsuspected condition will be identified. Balance testing also helps to objectively document the nature and severity of the problem. For example, a problem in the brain may be identified that was not suspected on the clinical examination. This would lead to a more sophisticated evaluation by a neurologist. Another example would be the person who has lost most of the inner ear function from exposure to a toxic medication. Although this may be suspected from the clinical history and the office exam, measuring the degree of the inner ear damage in a laboratory setting may determine whether rehabilitation is likely to be successful as well as helping to determine what type of treatment should be considered.

Sometimes patients with dizziness are involved in Worker's Compensation cases, disability claims or even litigation. While they may have fairly significant and disabling symptoms, their appearance and other test results may suggest that nothing is wrong. In these cases, it's especially helpful to be able to provide objective evidence of disordered function in the balance system. This helps to guide the physician's testimony and the court's decision in such complex cases.

Eye Movement Testing

Most balance testing begins with a series of fairly simple tests that measure your ability to control your eye movements. The eyes are controlled by the brain's signals to the muscles that move the eyeball. This process is called

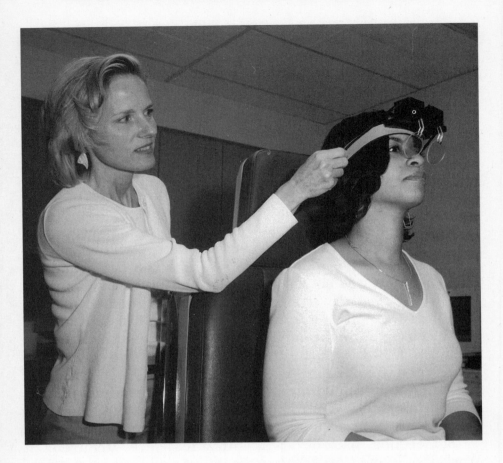

Figure 3-1: These unusual looking glasses are actually able to record eye movements of the patient during testing of the brain's ability to control eye movements and during a search for abnormal movements of the eyes (nystagmus) caused by disturbances in the vestibular system. After they are properly positioned and calibrated, the nature and speed of the eye movements can be recorded both on a video monitor and on a computer for precise analysis. This test is called *videonystagmography* which simply means using video techniques to record and analyze nystagmus. This system will eventually replace *electronystagmography,* a similar test that uses electrodes near the eyes instead of video goggles to record eye movements.

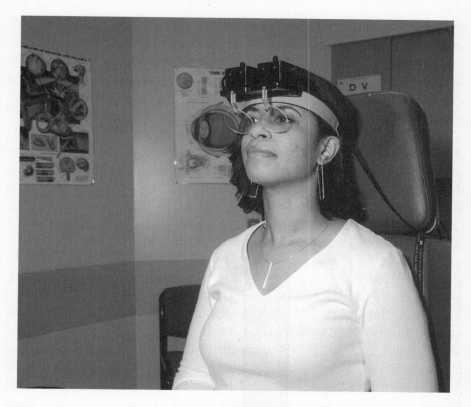

Figure 3-2: During videonystagmography, the patient is able to see clearly through the goggles during recording of eye movements. These goggles may also be used in darkness to record eye movements produced by irrigations that are designed to stimulate the inner ear by heating or cooling.

oculomotor control. Therefore, this portion of the assessment is sometimes called either "oculomotor testing" or "oculomotility testing." The name is not important. You should simply understand there are several very important functions that the eye and brain must be able to perform in a coordinated fashion, especially if you're performing complex balance tasks of any kind.

The testing begins by establishing a way to record the motion of the eyes (see Figures 3-1 and 3-2). This may be done by a video system or securing adhesive electrodes near the eyes that are able to sense eye movements. Historically, all balance testing labs used the electrode systems initially, but many programs are switching to systems using video recordings made by an infrared camera which allows us to see in the dark, much like the Army's night vision goggles. When such a system is in use, we may call the testing "videonystagmography."

In addition to avoiding electrode placements on the skin, these new systems allow video recording of the actual eye movements for review if needed during interpretation, which may be very helpful when questionable results are obtained. With conventional recording systems using electrodes, the patient would need to be called back to have the testing repeated in order to investigate any uncertainty in the original results. In very sophisticated research labs, search coils that are installed into contact lenses may be placed directly onto the eye.

Regardless of the method used, the first task will be to look at a red light positioned at a specific distance on either side of your head, and the equipment that measures the eye movement will be calibrated. This allows the ability to precisely measure the degree of eye motion during all the other tests. This data is recorded in a computer or, in older systems, on a strip of paper that is continuously feeding through a recording machine, much like an EKG for the heart or a lie-detector test.

Once eye movements are properly calibrated and being recorded, a series of eye movement tests are performed. The ability to locate and accurately look toward the red light (after it moves) is measured. As presented in Chapter 1, these sudden movements of the eye are called "saccades." We all use them every day to help orient us to our environment. Specific measurements of the time to onset of the saccade motion (latency), speed of the eye (velocity) and ability to hit the target without going past it (accuracy) are made. The results are compared to healthy individuals in your own age group. Delay in onset, slow maximum speed or inaccuracy of the movements suggest a problem in the brain's ability to control this type of eye movements.

Next, your ability to accurately follow a light that is moving predictably back and forth will be measured. This is called *smooth pursuit*, suggesting that the motion of the eye is expected to be smooth and consistent as it follows the target. Usually if the target movement is slow enough, the eye will track the light perfectly. As the speed increases, the eye may lag behind and have to make sudden movements (saccades) to catch up to the target. The older we become the harder this task is to perform. We expect the oldest patients to fail the test at the faster speeds, but the results are always compared to your own age group. The cerebellum is particularly important in smooth pursuit.

Lastly, the brain's ability to produce involuntary eye movements in response to a repeated motion in the visual environment is assessed. This is much like the balance system stimulation produced by looking out the side window of a car and watching trees go by—a common cause of motion sickness! The ability to produce this type of nystagmus is normal. It's also possible to increase the speed of the nystagmus as the speed of the visual stimulus increases. Failure to do so again suggests a problem within the brain.

Electronystagmography (ENG)

This test has a very intimidating name, but it basically means that we're going to measure the presence of nystagmus under a variety of testing conditions. In most clinics, everybody calls this test an "ENG," which is much easier to say. Usually when a doctor orders an ENG, it's assumed that both the oculomotor testing described earlier and the tests described in this section will be performed. That's because it is essential to know the status of the oculomotor control system in order to interpret the results of the rest of the ENG.

The ENG test begins with recording any eye movements while you are sitting still. It is important to remove any opportunity for vision during the ENG, since an individual will be able to suppress even fairly strong nystagmus by staring at an object in the room. (This normal function of the brain is called *visual fixation suppression*.) Therefore, the ENG test will be conducted either in darkness or with your eyes closed. There should not be any nystagmus noted whenever the head is still since the inner ears are not being stimulated. You may recall that a rhythmic eye movement seen in this neutral position is called spontaneous nystagmus. If spontaneous nystagmus is recorded and there were no abnormalities in the eye movement testing just described, it usually means that one of the inner ears and/or one balance nerve is sending the wrong signal into the brain. The exception to this rule would be when the nystagmus is vertical (beating up and down instead of side to side). Vertical nystagmus is a strong indication of a problem in the brain.

Then the examiner will look for nystagmus produced by changing the position of the head. This type of nystagmus is called *positional nystagmus* and tells us that the effects of gravity are not equal on both ears in various head positions. This is usually indicative of an inner ear problem. Sometimes we find there's no positional nystagmus in a particular position of the head unless the neck is also turned sharply in order to attain the position. This unusual finding suggests that the blood supply to the inner ear or brain is disturbed by the torsion of the neck. This may be an important indicator of insufficient blood flow in the vertebral arteries, which supply blood to the inner ear and parts of the brain most involved in balance control.

Sometimes the ENG battery includes a repeat of the Hallpike maneuver (previously described in the physical exam section) in an effort to record nystagmus associated with BPPV that might be produced by rapid changes in position of the head. Although this may be nice to document, the eye movement recordings may actually confuse the diagnosis since they usually come out opposite to the expected result. This is because it's difficult for the electrodes to detect rotation of the eyes and the recording system tells the computer that the eyes are beating in the direction opposite to what is observed when watching the eyes. The video system obviously would provide an opportunity to clarify this since the examiner can see the actual eye movements produced if the video is reviewed. However, just to make things simpler, I usually recommend that the examiner observe the eyes directly during the Hallpike maneuver rather than trying to record eye movements. In most cases of positional vertigo, the response to the movement is strong enough that visual fixation suppression will not occur.

The ENG concludes with the most memorable portion of balance testing: *caloric irrigations*. In this part of the test, the eye movements are recorded while stimulating the inner ears by changing their temperature. This is accomplished by the irrigation of warm and/or cool water into the outer ear canal. Water that is only 7° C (about 12.5° F) from body temperature will change the temperature of the inner ear sufficiently to provoke vertigo and nystagmus, assuming that both the inner ears and the balance nerves are healthy. Some labs use air irrigations or circulate the water inside little balloons placed in the ear canals in order to produce the responses. These are fine if good responses are produced, but the result is unreliable when poor responses are noted.

Our lab strongly prefers the instillation of water directly into the ear canal provided the eardrum is healthy. You should not allow water irrigation into your ear if you have an open mastoid cavity or if a perforation of the eardrum is known to be present. It's very important that the ear canals are clean prior to irrigation, since wax may block the water's entry inhibiting the heating or cooling effect deeper in the ear. This would give a false impression of an inner ear problem on that side. However, we do not recommend you personally try to clean out a wax blockage. The examiner should verify that the ears are open and that the canals are relatively symmetrical before performing the test. Even then, it's possible to gain a false impression of an inner ear problem if the technician does not perform equivalent irrigation procedures.

It is important to remember that it's normal to experience some vertigo during caloric testing. Some patients will experience nausea or other unpleasant symptoms in association with the vertigo, just as you may have experienced with your spells of vertigo. These feelings should pass fairly promptly.

Rarely, patients will become so sick that vomiting occurs. The technician is aware of this possibility and will be prepared to respond appropriately. Perhaps surprisingly, people with the most severe inner ear problems do not get very dizzy during the caloric test since their ears are unable to respond to the stimulus. In this case, sometimes ice water will be used to irrigate the ear in an effort to provoke a measurable response.

Usually caloric testing begins with warm water irrigation in one ear, the response is recorded and then the procedure is repeated in the other ear. If the nystagmus responses are equal or quite similar, it's not mandatory to perform cool irrigations. If one ear produces a much weaker response than the other, the technician will perform the cool water irrigations. The intensity of the response to each irrigation is measured and results for each ear are added together and compared to the other side's response. If one ear is more than 20-25 percent weaker than the other, we consider this to be abnormal, indicating a problem with the weaker ear or its nerve supply. This may be the only indication to tell us which ear is causing the dizziness you're experiencing, making this test extremely important.

It may also help to confirm a prior suspicion of a weak inner ear that was based on other symptoms, physical exam findings or the hearing test. In the case of an *acoustic neuroma* tumor (one that rises from the vestibular nerve that courses from the inner ear to the brain), the caloric test result may help the surgeon predict which nerve the tumor is arising from, as well as how dizzy you can expect to be after the tumor is removed. As in the other parts of balance testing, it's important not to become drowsy during the testing since this will suppress the nystagmus. This is not a problem if you're having a vigorous inner ear response, but if the ears are weak, the nystagmus may disappear if you start to drift off to sleep.

Therefore, the examiner may ask you to perform mental tasks to keep you alert, such as simple arithmetic problems or perhaps naming baseball teams, state capitols or U.S. presidents. If the examiner wishes to check out your ability to suppress nystagmus with visual fixation, the lights will be turned on briefly and you'll be asked to stare at a spot in the room. This will abruptly decrease the nystagmus until the lights are turned off again. Please recognize that although caloric irrigation may produce unpleasant symptoms, it often provides your doctor with the most important information needed to diagnose and treat your condition. For this reason, I find it very disappointing when a patient returns after testing and I'm told they either refused or could not complete the caloric testing.

In most clinical balance testing environments, the information gathered up to this point is all that can be acquired, due to limitations of space and the expense of the other testing equipment we will discuss next. Nonetheless, if there are definite abnormalities discovered on the ENG and eye movement testing, very important and specific conclusions may be made about the nature of your problem. In most clinics, this testing can be completed in about one hour. I would expect you to feel well enough to go home immediately. Usually, any unpleasant symptoms are limited to vertigo and nausea. These last for a few seconds up to a couple minutes in response to each caloric irrigation and pass quickly after the testing is completed. Because of the small chance of more extended nausea or vomiting in response to the caloric testing, you should not schedule another appointment right after your balance testing.

In all cases, I would advise you come accompanied by another individual who could drive you home after the testing if you don't feel well. Rarely a patient would need emergency treatment by a physician to help control nausea and vomiting. I have never had to admit a patient to the hospital for these symptoms. You should not hesitate to ask the testing personnel to assist you in receiving whatever care you need. All clinical labs have physician contacts for just this sort of problem and they'll know what to do to help you feel better.

Rotational Chair Testing

Although much useful information may be gained about the relative strength of the two inner ears from ENG testing, we must remember that our ears were not designed to respond to hot and cool water irrigation. This may go without saying, but it's appropriate to point out here that the inner ears are designed to respond to accelerations that are associated with movement of the head. Thus, a test that can objectively measure this type of normal physiologic response is highly desirable. *Rotational chair testing* was developed for just this purpose (see Figure 3-3). It involves the measurement of balance system responses to rotation of the head.

The actual phenomenon that is being measured has already been presented in Chapter 1—the *vestibulo-ocular reflex* or simply the VOR. You'll recall that the VOR functions primarily to stabilize the eyes so that you can continue to see clearly whenever your head is moving. In fact, it's these reflex movements that are being stimulated by water irrigations during the ENG.

The initial component of the eye movements that we call nystagmus is simply the normal eye motion provoked by the VOR. To put it simply, this is a reflex of the nervous system that causes the eyes to move in a very predictable way in response to stimulation of the inner ear balance system. Under normal daily conditions, each acceleration of the head produced by a rapid head movement is accompanied by an equal and opposite movement of the eyes that is almost instantaneous. This allows the visual environment to appear stable when we're moving about. When the balance system is disordered, abnormalities in the VOR function will produce dizziness and disorientation while you are active that may not bother you when your head is completely still. With *rotational chair testing*, we're going to look at the VOR responses to a more natural stimulus (controlled minor accelerations of the head) and we'll measure these responses at a variety of levels of stimulation.

The rotational chair test is performed with the patient in a motorized chair that calmly rotates back and forth. This test tells us how well the inner ears and brain perceive acceleration movements. It is performed in complete darkness so that there's no interference from the visual system. The camera is an infrared (night vision) video device that allows the examin-

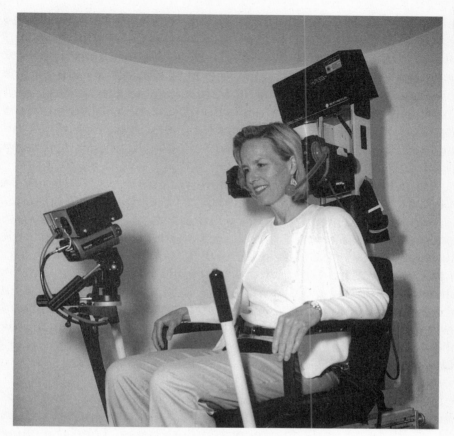

Figure 3-3: The Rotational Chair Test.

er to see the eye movements during testing, even in darkness. The head is tilted slightly down so the semicircular canals being tested will be truly horizontal in order to get the best responses.

The name "rotational chair testing" may evoke a somewhat foreboding sense of being spun dramatically in a chair as if at the local carnival. When you see the actual testing environment, your fears may initially increase. Why is this? The chair is centered in a fairly small and relatively soundproof chamber that allows for the testing to be conducted in darkness and quiet. As if that is not bad enough, the chair apparatus also includes straps for your body and a padded clamp that holds your head in place during the rotations. Some people with claustrophobia will be unable to coax themselves into the chair in the first place! But fear not. Once the testing actually begins, you'll realize it's really very safe and not particularly distressing. You'll be in constant contact with the technician by a simple intercom system, and an infrared camera system will allow the technician to monitor your face throughout the testing. Actually, the movements themselves are fairly modest, both in intensity and in ultimate velocity.

Rotational chair testing is performed for people who have special types of balance problems and for those whose problem cannot be confirmed using conventional ENG testing alone. It has been demonstrated that about one third of patients with dizziness whose ENG results are "normal" will have abnormalities confirmed by rotational chair testing. This unit is also particularly useful for testing infants and children who are too young to undergo caloric testing, and people who have lost function in both of their inner ears. The testing takes about 20-30 minutes and involves two basic testing procedures:

1. <u>Rotational Step Testing</u>: In this test, the chair is gradually accelerated to a constant velocity at which the VOR shuts off and the eye movements cease. Then the chair is rapidly stopped, which is a strong deceleration stimulus that will produce nystagmus. We can then record the strength and rate of decay of the nystagmus response. This is compared to normal values for people who do not have inner ear problems.

2. <u>Sinusoidal Harmonic Acceleration</u>: This test involves alternating slow chair accelerations and decelerations in a back and forth fashion. The alternating movements are performed at several frequencies that are slower than the average movements needed to fully activate the VOR in everyday life. This type of stimulation will expose VOR systems that are functioning abnormally. We can measure three different aspects of the VOR response.

- The first measurement is the ability of the VOR to produce an eye movement that is sufficient to stabilize the vision. This is calculated as a simple ratio of the size of the eye movement divided by the size of the head movement. The ratio is referred to as the "gain" of the response. Gain is typically lower than normal only if both inner ears are weak.
- The timing relationship of the eye movement to the head movement that stimulates it is very predictable. We call this measurement "phase" and can compare the phase of your VOR responses to normal individuals across a range of frequencies. If the VOR is not functioning correctly, the phase is usually abnormal in the low frequency range of testing.
- The strength of the eye movements produced by acceleration to the right can be compared to those produced by acceleration to the left. If these are not identical, as they should be, we can diagnose that an "asymmetry" is present in the response.

It is not generally possible to gain specific enough information from rotational chair testing to make a diagnosis of the cause of a vestibular problem. The noteworthy exception is when we're able to confirm bilateral loss of vestibular function. In other words, we may find that there is no VOR response or at least abnormally low gains throughout the testing. In these cases, we may be able to confirm that an antibiotic known to be toxic to inner ear function has indeed damaged the ears, or that a child with poor balance may have been born without adequate inner ear function.

Using rotational chair findings to support a diagnosis of inner ear malfunction may be helpful in documentation when the ENG is relatively normal. Unfortunately, it's impossible to say which ear is responsible for asymmetric responses. One ear may be underactive in stimulating the VOR or the other may be overactive. But we do know that most inner ear disturbances cause underactive responses. If the caloric response is also weak in the suspected ear, an asymmetry in the rotational chair test confirms that this weakness is producing an ongoing problem during head movement. After an individual compensates for the loss of balance function in one ear, the asymmetry will often resolve even if the caloric weakness is demonstrated to persist.

Rotational testing systems are very expensive, costing over $100,000 just for the chair itself and much more to outfit the lab space and install the system. The cost is prohibitive to most balance disorder programs in private offices and community hospitals, but increasingly these systems are available somewhere nearby in most regions of the country. Some balance testing labs have begun to use simpler (and much less expensive) systems to measure rotational responses such as the *Vestibular Autorotation Test* (VAT). This test involves acceleration sensors strapped to the head after which the patient is instructed to rotate the head side to side (or up and down) in time with an increasingly fast clicking sound. The apparatus can measure the gain of the VOR response over a range of frequencies that are important in everyday life and compare your responses to normal individuals.

Dynamic Posturography

The tests discussed so far have stressed measurement of the nervous system's ability to control eye movements and the responsiveness of the VOR to a variety of stimuli. Although these results may be very useful in detecting malfunctions in the vestibular system, none of these actually correlate with or really measure the ability of the individual to maintain balance. Some people may have very normal test results yet be extremely impaired in daily activities.

On the contrary, although this is less likely to be true, people with very abnormal ENG and rotational chair results may be perfectly functional when it comes to balance tasks. In an effort to specifically measure the stability of patients, many testing facilities have incorporated postural control assessments of some kind. These may involve measurement of performance on simple balance tasks as discussed in the physical examination section above, or may involve the use of sophisticated (and again expensive) equipment to measure postural control abilities.

The most commonly used equipment of this type is the EquiTest® system designed for a battery of tests known as *dynamic posturography*. This name simply means that there's a mechanism for measuring postural stability under various dynamic (changing) conditions. The equipment produces predictable challenges to the balance system and then measures how well the individual responds and maintains upright balance compared to other people their own age. The primary measurement tool is a movable force plate that the patient stands on. This force plate is able to sense the location of the individual and record the force generated by each foot in response to balance challenges (see Figures 3-4 and 3-5).

Platform posturography objectively measures the function of the entire balance system. The patient stands on a force-plate that is able to measure the sway of the body during testing, as well as the forces that are generated when responding to challenges to the balance system. The force-plate can also move or tilt suddenly to test the patient's ability to respond to a sudden disturbance of their balance. The contribution of the patient's visual system to their balance ability can be assessed by allowing movements of the large picture that surrounds them during testing.

Figure 3-5 shows the posturography unit during testing. The patient is secured in a safety harness similar to a parachute harness. This prevents any risk of falling during testing. The attendant is also close at hand to give instructions and reassure the patients regarding their safety.

The two primary components of the testing will be discussed here, although there are variations of commercially available equipment and testing protocols depending upon the needs and budget of the testing facility.

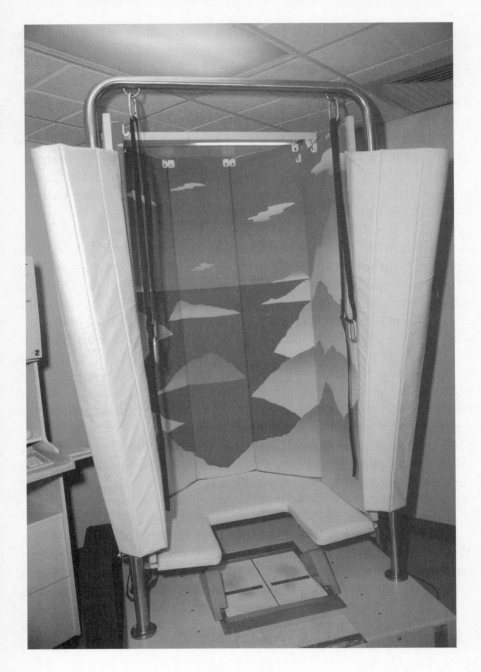

Figure 3-4: Testing Apparatus For Platform Posturography

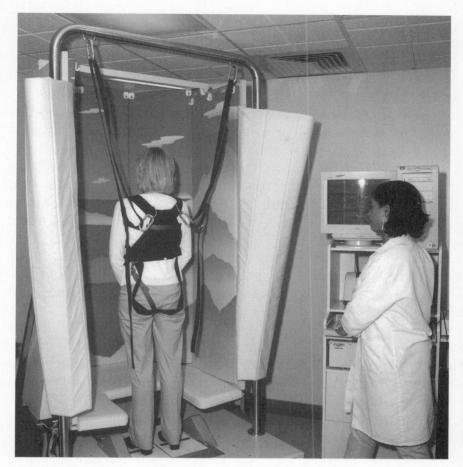

Figure 3-5: Posturography Unit During Testing

1. The Sensory Organization Test

This test measures your stability under several test conditions. You'll begin with a very simple task, but subsequent trials will be much more challenging. You may expect to be strapped into a safety harness similar to a parachute harness to prevent a fall if you lose your balance. The test technician should be nearby to assist you at all times as well. You'll step up onto the stable force plate and will be looking at a stable picture that fills your visual environment. If you're looking straight ahead you should not be able to see anything other than the picture even in your peripheral vision.

You'll be asked to stand completely still for 20 seconds. If you're very stable and your weight is evenly distributed on both feet, your result will look like equivalent flat lines for each foot. If you're swaying a lot, the lines will wobble dramatically. The computer then calculates the amount of sway as a percentage of perfect balance and gives a score.

For this first test condition, even people with balance problems usually score fairly well. If your score is poor and the examiner thinks it may be because you're nervous about the unfamiliar testing environment, the first test condition will be repeated.

Next you'll be asked to maintain your balance with your eyes closed. This is harder, especially for people who are relying on their vision because they have lost inner ear function.

The third test condition provides a more unique challenge and exploits a very useful function of the test equipment. In this test, you'll be asked to stand still again, but whenever you sway forward or back the visual surroundings will sway with you. Since this is (or should be) all you can see, even though you have your vision available to you, it's inaccurate and not helpful for maintaining your balance. We call this "sway-referenced vision." People who are overly dependent on their vision will become very unstable or even fall on this condition. However, this test is amusing but not difficult for people who have normal inner ear function and normal sensory function in their feet and legs.

After these three test conditions are scored, the same three tests are repeated with a little twist just to make it more interesting. The next time through (condition #4), the force plate that you're standing on will also be "sway-referenced." This means that whenever you tilt, the floor you're standing on will tilt with you. So, although your feet are still sending information to your brain about the floor beneath you, this is no longer accurate. If your vision is good and you're able to choose to use it for proper orientation, you'll be quite stable.

However, people who are depending on information from pressure sensors in their feet and stretch sensors in their ankles will become quite unstable.

When you're asked to either close your eyes (condition #5) or depend on vision that is also sway-referenced (condition #6), you'll be highly dependent on your inner ear function. If your ears are not normal you'll probably flunk the last two test conditions. This test helps your doctor and vestibular therapist understand what parts of the balance system are working properly, what parts of the system you're tending to rely upon for balance in challenging environments, and how stable (or unstable) you really are. It may also help determine what treatment the therapist will prescribe for you so that you're concentrating your efforts by doing those exercises that you need the most.

It's important to give your very best effort on the test. If you think your performance was poor due to nervousness and over-reactions, ask to try again. Some people who are trying to prove that they have a balance problem will attempt to appear worse than they really are when performing this test. This is actually quite foolish, since it's impossible to outwit the equipment. A sophisticated interpreter of the test results will recognize that you've been faking and will expose this in the report. If this occurs, it may diminish the credibility of any subjective symptoms you are reporting to the doctor. That in turn may actually hurt your claim for medical disability or any other monetary compensation that you may deserve for your balance system injury. However, I would stress that giving your best effort will produce a very accurate assessment of your balance system. This will be useful in counseling you about your problem, providing treatment and guiding legal testimony on your behalf if necessary.

2. Movement Coordination Test

This test measures the involuntary responses of the balance system to things that disrupt your balance. While you're standing on the support surface, the machine will suddenly move the force-plate a small degree forward or backward. The force plate measures the quickness, strength and accuracy of your response to the size of the movement that perturbed your balance. Slightly larger movements are then provided and the responses should increase appropriately.

Once this is completed, the test will be performed again, this time tilting the toes up or down. Even if the examiner tells you what will happen, the responses are automatic and not really under your voluntary control. So all you need to do is try to keep standing upright, no matter what happens to you. The information from this test is mostly helpful in sorting out whether there are any deficiencies in the sensory systems that inform the nervous system what has happened, or in the automatic muscle responses that the system produces.

Since the force plate is able to measure both feet independently, it can tell us whether you are supporting yourself with each foot equally. If you're using one foot primarily to stabilize yourself when your balance is disturbed, the machine will sense this also. The results may be impacted by joint problems in the leg or by spine problems. Since this part of the testing does not depend upon the inner ear, this test is not always performed when testing patients who are believed to have an inner ear disturbance.

Integration of Test Results
and Limitations of Balance Testing

Please remember what I stressed early in this chapter: With rare exceptions, the balance tests will not tell your doctor what the diagnosis of your condition is. There's only one test result that provides an exact diagnosis. That is the finding of a very specific abnormal eye movement result (called *internuclear ophthalmoplegia*) which is only seen in multiple sclerosis. But what sort of information may be gained in the average case? How are the tests useful?

Documentation of abnormalities: Many patients with vestibular disorders have significant symptoms and yet their physical examinations may be completely normal. When abnormalities are identified by balance testing, it helps the doctor to document objective physical problems that require further evaluation or treatment. On the other hand, sometimes a lack of abnormalities is helpful. For example, if someone has clear-cut symptoms and examination findings suggesting BPPV, it's helpful to find that there are no other abnormalities in the balance system. Then we can get right to treating the BBPV instead of doing lots of other testing. Likewise, if the exam and the balance tests are all completely normal, the doctor may determine that something unrelated to the balance system is causing the symptoms: perhaps hypoglycemia, migraine or an anxiety disorder.

Documentation of the site of the abnormality in the balance system: When the testing suggests there are abnormalities in the VOR but eye movement testing is normal, the problem must be located either in one of the inner ears or in the balance nerve that brings its signal to the brain. Unfortunately, both the ENG and the rotational chair only evaluate one of the three semicircular canals and its nerve supply. However, we know that it's rare for one isolated portion of the inner ear to be afflicted by anything that would cause dizziness without causing al least some disturbance in the rest of the inner ear. If the VOR testing is completely normal, but there are documented abnormalities in the oculo-motor test results, we suspect a problem somewhere in the brain. At times, the pattern of the abnormalities may point very clearly to one specific portion of the brain.

Documentation of which inner ear is affected: When the doctor is considering treatment of an inner ear condition that is not accompanied by hearing loss or other auditory symptoms, it is essential to document which ear is to blame. We also need to be sure not to carelessly suggest any surgery or other treatment that might injure inner ear function if the other ear's function was previously absent. Since rotational chair testing and posturography are testing both ears simultaneously, we still depend on the caloric irrigation results to tell us which ear has been damaged. An asymmetry on rotational chair testing may confirm our impression, but should not be used alone to make this judgment. Again, balance testing may allow your doctor to know for certain that your problems are related to the right inner ear, but this does not mean he will be able to tell you exactly why that ear is malfunctioning.

Documentation of bilateral loss of inner ear function: Some people will lose the function in both inner ears gradually in a very subtle fashion. This may occur rather suddenly from meningitis or more gradually while being treated with potentially toxic antibiotics for a serious infection elsewhere in the body. Symptoms may be severe but also very vague, so the diagnosis may be overlooked for quite some time. If caloric responses are reduced on the ENG, especially if the weakness persists even using ice water irrigations, a bilateral loss should be suspected. Such people should be referred for rotational chair testing to determine the severity of the loss, since this impacts their prognosis. They must also receive counseling about safety issues to prevent falling.

Documentation of vestibular compensation status: As discussed in Chapter 1, vestibular compensation is the process that the nervous system undergoes to recover from a prior vestibular system injury. Most of the patients that I am asked to evaluate for chronic balance problems continue to have symptoms due to delayed or incomplete compensation. Signs of incomplete compensation include persistent spontaneous or positional nystagmus, nystagmus after head shaking, rotational chair asymmetries, and certain abnormalities on posturography. These findings suggest that a course of vestibular rehabilitation may be helpful and some of the findings (posturography in particular) may help the therapist design the exercise program. However, if there are no abnormalities in the testing to suggest poor vestibular compensation, then I have to assume that there's some other inner ear problem. In this case, treatment is geared toward medical or surgical treatments to stabilize inner ear function. If this cannot be achieved, sometimes we'll choose to destroy the function in the unstable inner ear. That type of treatment will be discussed later in the book.

Summary

It is my hope that this chapter has prepared you for a favorable interaction with both your physician and the vestibular testing environment. Now you are armed with the type of information that will help you to anticipate what is going to take place and why it is being done. Hopefully you also have a good understanding of the complexities of the process and the uncertainties that your doctor faces every day.

Remember that the vestibular system is one of the more complex portions of the nervous system, and once it's injured it may not be possible to restore you to completely normal function. However, the vestibular system also has a remarkable propensity to adjust after an injury, provided that the inner ear function is either already stable or that the doctor can stabilize it for you. Vestibular rehabilitation may also play an important role in your treatment and offers you a great opportunity to actively participate in your own recovery.

CHAPTER FOUR

Medical Conditions Causing Dizziness

Glenn Johnson, MD

Associate Professor of Clinical Surgery at Dartmouth Medical School, Hanover, NH

Dr. Johnson is well-known for his expertise in the diagnosis and management of vertigo. He has made particularly important research contributions in the area of medical and surgical treatment for vertigo. He obtained his medical doctorate from George Washington University and did his otolaryngology surgical residency at Hershey medical Center in Pennsylvania. He did a fellowship in otology and neurotology with the Otology Group in Nashville, Tennessee. He has made many community and academic contributions serving on advisory boards, societies, and working as associate Professor of Clinical Surgery at Dartmouth medical school in Hanover, New Hampshire.

Dizziness can be caused or aggravated by a large variety of medical conditions and medications. General levels of strength, physical conditioning and activity levels will affect the degree of dizziness that is experienced, whatever the underlying cause. Even when the onset of dizziness can be clearly attributed to a very specific cause such as an *acoustic neuroma* the intensity, duration and disability caused by the sensation of dizziness can be modified by medical conditions. Unless recognized and managed, these medical issues can prevent the success of what otherwise would be an appropriate treatment program. In an attempt to simplify this complex area, it's helpful to review some basic concepts of the physiology of postural stability.

Our sense of balance (how stable we are in a variety of situations) is a very unique sense. As opposed to the senses of sight, hearing, touch, smell and taste, balance requires an integration of information from multiple sensory inputs: vestibular input from the inner ear, perception of movement perceived from vision and sensation of movement in our joints from *proprioception* (see Chapter 1). There's no such thing as a universal sense of balance that is true and accurate in all conditions. Each of the three senses that we (or more accurately our brains) use to give us a perception of where our body is in space and how fast we're moving is in relation to something else.

The inner ear relies on a change in head movement. The fluids of the semicircular canals obey the laws of physics and tend to stay put when the head is suddenly moved. This causes a deflection of the nerve endings in those semicircular canals which the brain uses to calculate speed and direction of head movement. A change in movement or acceleration of the head is needed to cause a movement of the skull in relation to the fluid in the semicircular canals. If the head and semicircular canal fluids are moving at the same speed (there is no acceleration), the inner ear perceives no movement. A simple example of this is traveling in your car at a steady rate of 65 miles per hour. Obviously, you're moving at a very fast speed, but the ear cannot perceive this since there's no acceleration.

Vision uses a different perspective for its relativity. We rely on seeing our head move in relation to objects that we can see to judge direction and speed of movement. When objects are close by, large and motionless, this sense is wonderfully accurate. If objects are far away and thus harder to see, this sense does not work as accurately. If all the objects around us are moving (such as when walking in a crowded shopping mall) our brain would need to calculate how fast we're moving in relation to many moving objects. This is too complicated to work well and in this situation vision is less helpful.

Proprioception perceives the relation of one part of our body to another, especially in the joints. It also perceives the pressure transmitted to our feet from the surface we are standing on. Proprioception tells our brain when the center of gravity of our body moves over our toes or from the left leg to the right. Neck proprioceptive fibers help the brain calculate how fast our head is rotating relative to the shoulders. Proprioception gives lots of input when lying in bed. Our entire body surface feels the contact of the bed from our feet to our head and uses this sense to tell if we're moving relative to that bed surface. When sitting in a comfortable chair, we feel through proprioceptive fibers the contact of our bottom and back against the chair. If there's no movement relative to the chair, we feel stable. Standing or walking uses fewer proprioceptive fibers (just the feet) and so gives less input. When walking on uneven ground, there's no reliable reference surface (as opposed to a flat even surface) rendering this sense of little value.

All these senses (and the brain) that need to blend the information into a single perception of movement and postural stability are affected by a variety of medical conditions. The brain is a crucial element in the sense of balance. It needs a certain critical amount of information from these three senses to feel confident in our stability. When these senses don't give enough information, the brain can not tell accurately how fast we are moving or where our body is in relation to our environment. We perceive this lack of accurate information as dizziness. When our brain is getting accurate information from two of the three senses, it is generally sufficient to produce a feeling of good balance. If however only one sense is working accurately, that will result in the feeling of imbalance, often to the degree that will cause a fall. Thus, a person with an inner ear cause of dizziness (Ménière's disease) will have a much more difficult time if they also have a medical condition that affects proprioception, for example, diabetes mellitus. With one sense that is malfunctioning (ear) and another that is not as sensitive as it should be (proprioception), accurate visual information is much more critical.

The evaluation of dizziness due to or aggravated by medical conditions follows the same systematic approach as the work-up of dizziness due to any cause. The history is the most critical piece of information. When vertigo develops suddenly without any precipitating movement, the cause is usually a sudden change in the information that the brain receives from the inner ear. The problem could be with the vestibular system in the inner ear or the neural connections between the ear and the brain.

Vision is affected by many medical conditions, but dizziness rarely if ever develops due to vision problems alone. If, however, you have poor vestibular and proprioceptive function, good vision is necessary to provide accurate information. If you need to wear bifocals and therefore cannot see the ground clearly when looking down through the bifocals, vision is less helpful when walking. Visual problems then may aggravate feelings of unsteadiness if there's a problem with the other balance senses.

Proprioceptive senses, especially in the feet, are affected by poor circulation to the lower legs and feet. The sensitivity of the proprioceptive input from the feet is also affected by neurological conditions such as peripheral neuropathies. If vision and vestibular function are good, a decrease in the proprioceptive sense causes subtle if any problems. But if the vestibular system is malfunctioning and/or vision is affected, poor proprioceptive input can cause a great deal of unsteadiness when walking.

Medical conditions that cause malfunction of brain function will affect balance in almost any conceivable way. When the character of dizziness does not follow any of the patterns typical for malfunction of the inner ear, vision or proprioception, abnormal brain function needs to be considered.

Some medical conditions that affect dizziness can be effectively treated. If cataracts are limiting vision, successful removal of the cataracts can have a significant benefit. Other medical conditions need to be controlled to minimize progression. Typical examples would be diabetes mellitus and peripheral vascular disease. The effects on the balance system by many medial conditions cannot be corrected. Treatment is by a vestibular rehabilitation approach that works to improve the brain's ability to use the senses that work and accommodate for the senses that do not.

Aging and Degenerative Processes

Aging has many potential effects on the sense of balance. A decrease in the acuity of many of our senses is a very common, although not universal part of aging. Gradual loss of hearing especially in the higher frequencies is so common as we age that it's given the term *presbycusis*. Although it's difficult to prove, some decrease in the sensitivity of the balance system in the inner ear probably occurs to some degree with aging. Loss of visual acuity is also common. It may be limited to difficulty reading at close distances or present with more severe problems due to the development of cataracts or macular degeneration. Decreased circulation to the feet is also common due to atherosclerotic vascular disease (commonly referred to as hardening of the arteries: *atherosclerosis*). This decreased blood supply may be accompanied by a decreased sensation to touch on the soles of the feet. This makes it harder to sense our body shifting to one foot or from our toes to our heels. A decrease in the sensitivity of any one sense of balance decreases the sharpness or sensitivity of our stability. If two or even three of these senses lose some sensitivity, it can have a more significant effect on our sense of stability.

As we age, most of us tend to get more cautious. We realize that we heal more slowly from even minor injuries. *Osteoporosis* (reduced bone density causing brittle bones) is another common condition that accompanies aging especially in women. Falls are therefore more likely to result in bone fractures. The consequence of fearing falls is that older individuals are more likely to cut back on activity as a result of feeling unsteady. Rather than do challenging activities to strengthen the balance system, the unsteady older individual commonly cuts back on walking trips outside. Outdoor activities that involve complex head and body movements are substituted for more sedate activities indoors. As a result of decreased activity, the balance system gets less exercise. It gets out of shape so to speak. With less training, less stimulation, the instability gets worse. This causes a further cut-back in activity and the instability gets even worse. As you can see from this progression, symptoms of unsteadiness can be aggravated by decreasing activity as a result of caution and a fear of falling.

A further aggravating factor that typically occurs with aging and a decrease in activity is a decrease in muscle strength, especially in the legs. A young healthy athlete who is put on bed rest for only a few weeks will lose a substantial amount of muscle mass in the quadriceps muscle, the major muscle in the thigh. Almost everyone loses some muscle mass and strength with aging, and this is significantly accelerated by a decrease in activity, primarily weight bearing activity such as walking. Muscle strength and flexibility are a critical part of our postural stability. If the small movements that occur while merely standing still are analyzed, the role of our leg muscles will become clear.

Nobody is perfectly still while standing. Our body moves slowly from side to side and from front to back to such a subtle degree that we're not even conscious of it. As our body moves to the right, proprioceptive fibers sense an increase in pressure on the right foot and decrease in pressure on the left foot. This causes a reflex increase in the tone of the extensor muscle in the right leg (the muscle that causes the leg to push toward the floor). If the muscle is strong it will very effectively change the direction of body sway and push it gently back toward the center. The body then sways toward the left and the same thing happens. Front to back movement is controlled by the calf muscles that push the toes and balls of the feet down to move our body backwards and a relaxation of these same muscles when our body moves too far toward our heels.

Now let's go through the same sway with weaker muscles. As our body movement sways toward the right foot, the extensor muscles start to contract. A weak muscle will not be very effective in slowing down the movement toward the right and our body continues to sway more to the right. Before long, our body sway has moved so far to the right that the weak muscles can no longer hold it up and we fall. The leg muscles may not be part of the balance sensory system, but they play a very important part of keeping our body upright and centered over our two feet. Lower extremity (thigh and calf) strengthening exercises usually involving weight or resistance exercises almost always improves the stability in an older person, regardless of the cause of the unsteadiness.

Atherosclerosis and Hypertension

Elevated blood pressure (*hypertension*) rarely would be considered to be the underlying cause of symptoms of dizziness. Hypotension, however, can cause a very characteristic pattern. This entity referred to as *postural hypotension* produces symptoms of dizziness with a change of body position from lying down to sitting, or lying or sitting to standing. The arteries (those vessels that carry blood from the heart to muscles and organs of our body) have a layer of smooth muscle in the arterial wall. This allows the arteries to enlarge or contract in order to regulate the proper flow of blood to the tissue that the arteries supply. When we're lying flat in bed, it's very easy for the heart to pump blood to the brain because it doesn't have to pump against gravity. Therefore, when lying down, the artery wall is relaxed and the opening is large to allow an easy flow of blood.

When we stand up quickly, suddenly the heart has to pump blood against gravity. The muscles in the artery wall suddenly contract helping to force the blood up to the brain. An analogy would be a balloon full of water. If you squeeze the balloon the water will squirt out the opening. If the artery walls constrict too slowly or not at all, the blood will take more time to get up to the brain. This few second delay in getting sufficient blood to the brain decreases the amount of oxygen available for brain function. This lack of sufficient oxygen causes the feeling of faintness.

The feeling that develops from a brief period of too little oxygen to the brain causes several symptoms. Often the first is a sense of lightheadedness. A perception of whirling vertigo is not usually experienced. Vision typically gets fuzzy or blurry. The leg muscles feel weak. If the brain goes for more than a few seconds without adequate oxygen, we faint. The treatment is to lay down allowing an easy flow of blood that doesn't have to work against gravity. Since the symptoms of postural hypotension are caused by low oxygen to the entire brain, other symptoms in addition to lightheadedness are always experienced. Fuzzy, blurred or darkened vision is the most common additional symptom experienced.

There are many causes of postural hypotension. Some young healthy people who have low normal blood pressure will experience this symptom very briefly when going quickly from laying down to standing. Many medications that work to lower high blood pressure decrease the muscle tone in the arterial walls and as a result increase the likelihood of postural hypotension. Dehydration can contribute to this symptom by lowering blood volume.

Fainting Spells

Common fainting spells are most commonly caused by an error in the autonomic nervous system. It occurs when the system misinterprets blood flow the body needs while standing upright and sending the wrong message to the heart and blood vessels, causing the heart to slow down and the blood pressure to fall. Long periods of standing, exercise and exposure to warm temperatures typically bring on this condition. As a result of this drop in blood flow to the brain, sufferers feel lightheaded, occasionally accompanied by nausea, and feel like they're going to faint. Some may actually fall, but usually sitting or lying down will allow this sensation to pass. For some people with this condition, a feeling of tiredness or lethargy may persist for several days after such an incident.

Common fainting spells are also known by other names: neurocardiogenic *syncope*, neurally mediated syncope, vasodepressor syncope, vaso-vagal syncope and neurally mediated hypotension. Normally, our blood pressure is regulated by the autonomic nervous system to respond to different stresses. This complex set of nerves changes the blood flow to our brain and other organs depending on their oxygen needs. If we're exercising, blood flow is diverted to our muscles. After eating, blood flow is preferentially sent to our stomach and intestines to digest the food. These changes in blood flow are accomplished by changing the rate of contraction of the heart, changing the strength of heart contraction and changing the diameter of the blood vessels supplying the different organs of our body.

Neurocardiogenic syncope cannot be diagnosed by checking your pulse or blood pressure during a routine physical exam. It is diagnosed by a specific study known as a "tilt table test," typically performed by a cardiologist. The tilt table test goes through a specific protocol to evaluate how the blood pressure and heart rate respond to changes in body elevation. People tolerate this test very well. Nevertheless, for safety, an intravenous line (a needle placed in the vein) is maintained in case you feel faint during the test.

The exact protocol for this test may vary to some degree, but usually proceeds along the pattern described here. The table is tilted so your head is elevated 30°. Blood pressure and heart rate are evaluated in this new position for about five minutes. If there's no significant change, the table is tilted further so the head is elevated 60°. Blood pressure and heart rate are usually monitored for up to 45 minutes in this position, since with neurocardiogenic syncope, it can take up to 30 minutes or longer for an inappropriate drop in blood pressure to occur.

If there is no abnormality noted this far, the table is placed flat again and a drug similar to adrenaline is injected through the intravenous line. The drug often used is Isoproterenol (Isuprel™), and is similar to what your own body produces during times of exercise or stress. The table is again tilted to 60 degrees and kept at this level for about 15 minutes. An abnormal (positive test) occurs when a drop in blood pressure occurs associated with symptoms of lightheadedness, nausea, sweating, a cold clammy feeling or the sensation of fainting.

Treatment for neurocardiogenic syncope is not universally agreed upon. It may include efforts to increase fluid and/or salt intake. Medications that regulate blood pressure may be used as well as drugs that block the body's response to adrenaline. Specific treatment will depend on the individual's personal medical history, test results and the experience of the treating cardiologist.

Neurocardiogenic syncope may cause dizziness but does not cause other ear symptoms such as hearing loss, tinnitus or ear fullness. Lightheadedness occurs almost exclusively in the standing position; and prolonged standing, exercise or stress, or rapidly sitting up may be contributing factors. The tilt table test may be abnormal, but all other diagnostic tests should be normal.

Cardiac

A sudden change in the effective pumping of the heart is another cause for a decrease in oxygen supply to the brain. Postural hypotension is usually brief, brought on in a very repeatable pattern of a change in posture from lying or sitting to standing and almost always corrects itself within a few seconds.

In contrast, hypotension can occur at any time even without a position change, if there's a problem with the heart. A decrease in heart-pumping efficiency may cause a dramatic drop in oxygen delivery to the brain. The result is often a sudden loss in stability and loss of consciousness (*syncope*). Someone who has experienced syncope simply finds themselves on the ground without the clear recollection of how they got there. They may recall suddenly becoming light-headed or feeling faint but they have no conscious recollection of the exact events that lead to a fall to the ground. The conscious reflex to protect oneself during a fall is lost, so an injury to the head or body is not uncommon during the syncopal episode. The loss of consciousness, even for a brief second, can never be attributed to abnormal inner ear function. (There have been very rare cases in which syncope, a fainting spell, occurred with a profoundly strong vertigo attack from the inner ear. The vaso-vagal reaction to the vertigo attack caused the syncope, not the inner ear itself. Whenever there is a true loss of consciousness, it cannot be blamed on the inner ear and must be thoroughly investigated—Ed.)

The most common cardiac cause for syncope is an abnormal heart rhythm called an arrhythmia. This might be diagnosed by feeling the pulse. Normally one's pulse should have a regular pattern. If the pulse occasionally skips a beat or feels generally irregular it could represent a chronic arrhythmia. A more formal way to diagnose irregularities of cardiac rhythm is with an electrocardiogram (ECG). Other cardiac arrhythmias occur suddenly and infrequently. The short few minutes it takes to perform an ECG may not be long enough to pick this up. A *holter monitor* is a portable ECG monitor that is typically worn for 24 hours. When symptoms of lightheadedness are felt, the wearer pushes a button on the monitor. If an irregular heartbeat is seen at the time that lightheadedness was experienced, it strongly suggests that the cardiac irregularity was the cause of the lightheadedness.

Abnormal cardiac rhythms can be caused by problems in many different areas of the rhythm-generating system in the heart. Diagnosis is best made by a physician (with experience in heart diseases) following appropriate diagnostic tests. Treatment may involve medications, use of an electrical discharge to "shock" the heart into a more normal rhythm (electrical cardioversion) or the surgical placement of a mechanical device that electrically stimulates the heart at an appropriate rate (pacemaker).

Cerebrovascular: Vertebro-Basilar Insufficiency

A decrease in blood flow through narrowed blood vessels that supply the area of the brainstem containing the vestibular nucleus and neural projections to higher centers of the brain can cause temporary or permanent changes in those nerve pathways. The nerve fibers in the brain that carry information from the inner ear are supplied oxygen and nutrients by blood flow through the vertebral arteries. The two vertebral arteries that run on either side of the cervical spine merge together inside the skull to form one basilar artery. Multiple small branches of the basilar artery enter the brainstem to perfuse the many nerve tracts that course there, which include fibers supplying information from the inner ear.

The vertebral and basilar arteries, like most arteries in the body, can become narrowed by plaques of atherosclerosis. This narrowing can cause a decrease in blood flow and if decreased enough, a loss of function of the nerve tracts supplied by those vessels can result. If the nerve tracts affected are those from the inner ear, dizziness or vertigo can occur. But these blood vessels supply more nerve tracts in the brainstem than just those from the inner ear. Therefore, insufficient blood flow through the vertebro-basilar blood vessels or their tributaries causes a multitude of symptoms along with dizziness. Other typical symptoms can include clumsiness, weakness, paralysis, difficulty pronouncing words correctly, loss of vision or double vision. This relatively unique group of additional symptoms effectively separates dizziness due to vertebro-basilar insufficiency from many other causes.

Hyperlipidemia (Hypercholesterolemia)

Lightheadedness has been associated with marked elevations of the large fatty molecules, cholesterol and triglycerides. Why high levels of these substances cause dizziness is not clear, but a common theory is that they narrow the blood vessels that supply the inner ear and balance centers of the brain. Another concept is that because they are large molecules they thicken the blood (increasing viscosity) and make it more difficult to squeeze through the tiny capillaries that supply nutrients to these neural tissues. A fasting blood test (blood sampled after not eating food for 14 hours) for the lipids, cholesterol and triglycerides is the best way to test for this condition. Dietary changes and lipid-lowering drugs may cause an improvement in dizziness if effective in lowering the blood level of these substances.

Abnormal glucose (sugar) metabolism has also been thought to cause symptoms of dizziness. After food that contains glucose is absorbed into the bloodstream by digestion, insulin is necessary to allow that glucose to be transported into the cells. All tissues use glucose for fuel, but nerve tissue can only use glucose (not fat or protein) for its fuel source. If too much insulin is secreted by the pancreas for the amount of glucose that is in the bloodstream, too much glucose will be absorbed into the cells and glucose levels will drop too low. This condition (*hypoglycemia*) can cause dizziness or lightheadedness because the neural tissue of the brain does not get enough glucose to function normally. Hypoglycemia is diagnosed by a glucose tolerance test. A blood sample is analyzed for glucose after fasting. The patient then consumes a soda-like drink loaded with glucose. Following this, blood samples are taken for the next three to five hours to determine how high and then low the blood glucose levels go. Hypoglycemia is diagnosed if the blood glucose falls below around 60 mg/dl associated with symptoms of dizziness. Some experts in dizziness feel that a flat glucose tolerance curve (that is, very little elevation or drop in glucose levels during a five-hour glucose tolerance test) can also be associated with dizziness.

Treatment for hypoglycemia is by dietary management. Concentrated sugars and simple carbohydrates like donuts, sweets and starches are avoided since these foods allow a large sudden load of glucose to be absorbed. Instead, complex carbohydrates that need to be slowly broken down into sugars or proteins and fats are eaten. Many small meals instead of a few large meals will also lessen the likelihood of a quick rise and then fall in blood sugar levels.

Cervical Vertigo

The neck can play a significant role in causing or contributing to symptoms of dizziness or vertigo. Proprioceptive nerve fibers are present in abundance in the neck and vertebral joints of the cervical spine. These fibers (through the vestibulo-spinal tracts) join up with the nerves from the semicircular canals of the inner ear within the area of the brain known as the vestibular nucleus. Since so much of our daily activity involves moving the head from side to side, it's reasonable to theorize that the brain uses two simultaneous systems to track head movement: the vestibular system in the inner ear and proprioceptive fibers in the neck.

Proprioceptive fibers in the joints of the cervical vertebrae (the individual bones in the neck's backbone) relay the movement and position of the bony skeleton. Fibers in the neck muscles relay relative tone or tension of the muscles.

If the muscles on the right side of the neck are tighter than those on the left, this would normally indicate that the tighter right-sided muscles are pulling the head toward the left. For complex quick head movements, information from the vestibular system in the ear works with proprioceptive input from the neck to give us a very accurate sense of where our head is relative to our environment.

Since proprioceptive fibers from the neck relay information to the same area of the brain as the vestibular system in the ear, abnormalities of the neck causing vertigo can cause symptoms that are very similar, and often hard to distinguish from symptoms of dizziness caused by inner ear malfunction. An abnormal tightness of the neck muscles (a condition often referred to by the term myofascial pain) often causes referred pain or discomfort affecting the ear on that side.

Those afflicted with this condition will often describe a sense of fullness in the ear, a symptom that leads many to suppose the presence of fluid in the middle ear or the diagnosis of Ménière's disease. One very helpful clue is that hearing loss often accompanies inner ear malfunction such as Ménière's disease, but hearing loss never accompanies vertigo or dizziness caused by the neck. (Another hint is that cervical problems are usually made worse by prolonged head movement such as maintaining the neck turned to one side. Cervical vertigo will not usually cause the spontaneous or "out of the clear blue" unprovoked vertigo attacks seen in Ménière's disease and some other conditions. Any disequilibrium of any sort, including cervical vertigo, may cause some sensation of imbalance or brief vertigo with a rapid head movement.—Ed.)

Migraine

Dizziness and vertigo associated with migraine can present with a variety of symptom patterns. Although there are differences that will be detailed later in this section, the pattern of dizziness or vertigo may seem similar to what occurs in Ménière's disease, benign paroxysmal positional vertigo (BPPV) or vestibular neuronitis. Often migraine is considered as an underlying factor in the cause of dizziness only after repeated attempts to treat the dizziness as Ménière's disease or other suspected diagnoses have failed to give adequate control. The diagnosis of migraine-related dizziness is made by combining a detailed analysis of the history of the dizzy symptoms, the history of headaches in the person suffering from dizziness as well as in family members, evaluation of inner ear function by hearing tests and vestibular studies, and ruling out other disorders of the brain or central nervous system by exam and often imaging studies. Since there's no single diagnostic study that indicates migraine as the cause of dizziness, this diagnosis is difficult to distinguish from other entities that lack a well-defined gold standard test such as perilymph fistula.

Contrary to common perception, migraine is more than a headache disorder. Migraine is an inherited condition characterized by an abnormality in the part of the brain that regulates (actually suppresses) the intensity of sensory input. The sense usually thought of is pain or more specifically head or neck pain. But other senses are involved as well. Light is perceived as too bright; sound is too loud; and aromas are too overpowering. All this overemphasis of sensory input (hypersensitivity) is most pronounced during a migraine attack when the sufferer has a severe pounding headache combined with *photophobia* (light is too bright), *phonophobia* (sound is too loud) and nausea. But even between headache attacks, migraine sufferers typically find they cannot tolerate bright lights or loud sounds as comfortably as others can.

It is this hypersensitivity phenomena that is thought to be a major factor in the development of the symptoms of dizziness. Motion is perceived by several senses, specifically the inner ear, proprioceptive senses (with a large component in the neck) and vision. If the brain increases the perception of movement as sensed by the inner ear and/or neck to be greater than it really is, we perceive the sensation of dizziness, vertigo or motion sickness.

Migraine Diagnosis

Migraines produce characteristic headaches and other symptoms that help differentiate them from other types of headaches. A migraine headache is described by the International Headache Society as characterized by at least five attacks fulfilling A - C below:

A. Headache attacks lasting 4-72 hours (untreated or unsuccessfully treated)
B. Headache has at least two of the following characteristics:
   - unilateral location
   - pulsating quality
   - moderate or severe intensity (inhibits or prohibits daily activities) aggravation by walking stairs or similar routine physical activity
C. During headache at least one of the following:
   - Nausea and/or vomiting
   - Photophobia and phonophobia

Although there are many subtypes of migraine, the two most common are migraine with "aura" and migraine without aura. An aura is a temporary neurological symptom (usually a visual sensory abnormality such as flashing lights, wavy lines like oil slicks, or blind spots). Other sensory abnormalities such as numbness, tingling and vertigo may also occur. When auras occur they usually develop before the headache and the aura symptoms last from 5-60 minutes and completely go away. The headache then follows. Rarely, aura symptoms last for more than 60 minutes and then are classified as migraine with prolonged aura.

A less common form of migraine is one without a headache. In this migraine subtype, there are symptoms such as a typical migraine aura but without the headache that usually follows. Dizziness related to migraine may occur without any present or past history of headache.

Migraine-Related Dizziness and Vertigo

When dizziness occurs, how long it lasts and what brings it on varies from one migraine-related dizziness sufferer to another. There are, however, several patterns that can be described, but the most common three are cited below:

1. Vertigo as an Aura with Basilar Migraine

Basilar migraine has a particular type of aura that involves the senses that are supplied by the basilar artery. The aura usually includes visual symptoms noted in both eyes, ringing in the ears, muffled hearing, dizziness or vertigo and then numbness or tingling in the hands or feet. When dizziness is part of the aura, it typically lasts (like all aura symptoms) 5-60 minutes. The headache that follows is usually felt in the back of the head.

2. Benign Recurrent Vertigo

The vertigo that occurs in the pattern called benign recurrent vertigo is very similar to a subtype of Ménière's disease called vestibular Ménière's disease. In this entity, true spinning vertigo develops in a sudden, spontaneous fashion. The vertigo lasts hours to several days in duration. When it does last longer than 24 hours, this helps to distinguish it from Ménière's disease which rarely causes vertigo longer than one day. Often, brief vertigo is experienced after head movement for several days after a typical episode.

What distinguishes this entity from Ménière's disease is the absence of hearing loss. Tinnitus and fullness can be felt in one or both ears, but a significant loss of hearing does not occur. Hypersensitivity to loud sounds (phonophobia) is often described; a symptom characteristic of migraine.

The vertigo with benign recurrent vertigo typically does not occur with a headache. Often the sufferer had migraine-like headaches earlier in life and now just gets occasional headaches that may behave more like a tension headache than a typical migraine headache.

Distinguishing the vertigo of benign recurrent vertigo from Ménière's disease is often difficult. Spontaneous-occurring vertiginous spells that last several days in duration are probably not due to Ménière's disease. Vertiginous spells that last several hours and are associated with tinnitus and ear fullness could be early Ménière's disease or benign recurrent vertigo. Since Ménière's disease may present for months or even years with vertiginous episodes before the hearing loss develops, the distinction between the two may only be able to be made after observing for several years.

3. Migraine-Associated Vertigo

Dizziness and vertigo related to migraine can also occur in less well-defined patterns than that described with basilar migraine or benign recurrent vertigo. Symptoms can include a continuous feeling of unsteadiness, "motion intolerance" (dizziness or vertigo felt either when moving or seeing other objects moving), *positional vertigo* (vertigo experienced with change in position), or spontaneous episodes. The positional vertigo that occurs with migraine-related vertigo often develops with almost any head movement, not just the typical position changes seen in BPPV. Not infrequently, one person can have a combination of baseline unsteadiness, position-induced vertigo and spontaneous episodes of vertigo.

Diagnosis of Migraine-Related Vertigo

The headache that occurs with basilar migraine is characteristically at the back of the head and closely associated with the onset of the vertigo. Benign recurrent vertigo needs to be distinguished from early Ménière's disease because there may be little or no headaches. Over time it's usually possible to distinguish the two since hearing loss invariably occurs with Ménière's disease within a year or so.

For the less stereotypical patterns, several factors are usually necessary to make the diagnosis. These include: absence of a hearing loss by audiological testing, history of migraine-like headaches either presently or in the past, a family history of migraine (with or without headache), and exclusion of other diseases by history or testing. This last issue is critical. The pattern of dizziness should not be consistent with other clearly defined patterns of dizziness such as Ménière's disease, vestibular neuronitis or BPPV. There should be no suggestion of cardiac dysfunction or other neurological disease, and no indication of structural brain disease. Often, a brain MRI is necessary to exclude the later.

Diagnostic tests for migraine-related dizziness typically give either normal results or abnormalities seen with inner ear dysfunction. Hearing tests are almost always normal although there are occasional exceptions. ENGs are either normal or show abnormalities seen with peripheral disease such as caloric weakness or positional nystagmus. Platform posturography may be normal or show poor stability in the most challenging conditions (5 and 6) usually seen with peripheral dysfunction. The exam is usually normal, but may show tenderness with palpation (touching and feeling) of the upper neck muscles. There may be rotation when walking in place with the eyes closed (*Fukuda stepping test*).

The treatment for migraine-related dizziness optimally requires a combination of approaches. Foods linked with precipitating or causing migraine headaches should be avoided. These include caffeine, chocolate and the artificial sweetener aspartame or brand name Nutrisweet. Foods high in protein containing the amino acid tyramine should also be avoided. These include strong cheeses and red wine.

Balance therapy, typical to what is used to treat peripheral inner ear dysfunction with excessive reliance on visual input, is often very helpful. If neck muscle spasm and tenderness is present, often in a myofascial pain pattern, then physical therapy to the neck is beneficial. Lifestyle changes can help, primarily improved sleeping patterns and stress reduction. If all these measures are not successful in controlling the vertigo, then medication may be indicated.

Drugs used to treat migraine-related dizziness include several different classes of medications used as prophylaxis for migraine headaches. These include tricyclic medications such as amitriptyline and nortriptyline, calcium channel blockers, and selective serotonin reuptake inhibitors. Tricyclic antidepressants may be very effective in doses far below those used to treat depression. Calcium channel blockers are normally used for lowering high blood pressure or treating cardiac conditions, but again may work well for migraine treatment even in low doses.

These medications are typically chosen to decrease the frequency of spontaneous episodes of vertigo. The other classes of drugs used are benzodiazepines (anti-anxiety medications that can be effective also in low doses). These drugs enhance the major inhibitory neurotransmitter in the brain (gamma amino butyric acid—GABA). They probably work by decreasing the sensitivity of the motion sensors in the inner ear. Lorazepam (Ativan™), clonazepam (Klonopin™), and diazepam (Valium™) are the most commonly used drugs in this class.

Multiple Sclerosis

Multiple sclerosis (MS) is an autoimmune disorder that selectively destroys the myelin-insulating sheaths that surround individual nerve fibers in the brain, spinal tract and optic nerve. The damaged myelin sheaths are then replaced by scar tissue called plaques. This loss of effective insulating sheath causes the nerves to malfunction, similar to the short-circuiting that develops in an electrical wire if the insulating coating is worn off.

The symptoms that develop from MS result from the specific nerve tracts that are damaged. Unsteadiness or difficulty walking, numbness or "pins and needles" felt in the hands and feet, and visual loss are commonly experienced symptoms with MS. Tremor, slurred speech, difficulty swallowing, weakness of arms or legs, and loss of coordination also can occur. True whirling vertigo is relatively rare. The hallmark of MS is that these widely varied symptoms may occur simultaneously or at different times and clearly involve different unrelated areas of the brain. It's also common for these symptoms to come and go, with long periods of remission when the symptoms are completely gone.

There's no single test that will accurately diagnose MS. It takes a combination of: 1) a pattern of symptoms compatible with MS; 2) physical exam abnormalities that may include abnormal reflexes, vision, pinpoint and vibration sensitivity, and balance, and; 3) abnormal test results.

The most commonly used studies include nerve function testing of vision, hearing and sensation, analysis of the spinal fluid obtained from a spinal tap, and MRI scan of the brain and spinal column that shows areas of plaques.

Cerebrospinal fluid (CSF), the clear watery fluid that bathes and surrounds the brain and spinal cord, is tested for antibodies and proteins that result from the breakdown of the myelin sheath. An MRI scan can show very characteristic areas of demyelination in the brain that appear as white spots or streaks on a particular sequence (known as T2 weighted imaging).

One of the difficulties that can occur is that small white spots on T2 sequences of an MRI scan can occur in perfectly normal people. Specialists in neurology and "neuroradiology" (a radiologist who specializes in brain and spinal cord imaging) have developed criteria for these white spots to help differentiate "normal" from those that are strongly characteristic of MS. But it must be emphasized that MS cannot be diagnosed by just one abnormal test. The history, neurological exam and abnormal test results must be taken together in order to give the best ability to accurately diagnose this condition.

Medication

Medications can cause dizziness or lightheadedness, aggravate the intensity of dizziness from other causes, or prolong the recovery from a condition that causes dizziness. The same drug that may lessen the feeling of dizziness in one person may increase it in another. The same drug may help the dizziness in one stage of a disorder and make it worse in another. This is a complex and confusing area, but there are some basic concepts that will help you understand how medication can help or aggravate the sensation of dizziness.

Some drugs in and of themselves can cause dizziness. Types of drugs that can have this effect include:

- Drugs that are designed to change brain or neural function. These include drugs used to treat mood, emotional or psychiatric conditions, muscle relaxants, sedatives, pain killers, sleeping pills and antiseizure medications;

- Drugs that alter blood pressure, either as a side effect of the drug or when used to treat high blood pressure.

- Drugs that aggravate an existing condition that causes dizziness typically work as sedatives that reduce alertness and the coordination needed to compensate or adjust to dizziness. The trickiest group of drugs is generally prescribed to treat dizziness. These are usually antihistamines with some sedative effect, such as meclizine. Benzodiazepines such as diazepam and clonazepam are also used.

During the early stages of a condition characterized by severe, prolonged vertigo such as vestibular neuronitis, these drugs help reduce the intensity of the severe dizziness and help to minimize the resultant nausea and vomiting. After the severe stage is over, these drugs may prolong recovery by causing drowsiness which limits activity or by reducing the effectiveness of compensation by balance rehabilitation.

Scopolamine patches, also used to treat motion sickness or reduce the intensity of a severe attack may actually cause persistent dizziness if used for weeks or months on a continuous basis. A basic concept for optimal use of these drugs is to use them as directed by your physician when the intensity of the dizziness is so severe that you feel nauseated and cannot continue with relatively normal activity. When the dizziness has settled down to the point where you can "work through it," that is, it's bothersome and noticeable, but you can go on with life in spite of it, it is usually best to stop the drug. Clonazepam (a long acting, potent benzodiazepine) is often used to control long-term chronic dizziness. Going off this drug requires a gradual slow taper since dizziness can develop as a withdrawal symptom if it's stopped abruptly.

Conclusions

As you can see, the medical and neurological conditions that cause dizziness and vertigo are not simple issues to diagnose or treat. It will be important that you work with your physician and explain as best you can what your symptoms are and what patterns occur . This will be one of the most important tools by which your diagnosis is made.

References

1. Headache Classification Committee of the International Headache Society. Classification and diagnostic criteria for headache disorders, cranial neuralgias and facial pain. *Cephalgia* 1988;8:19-73.
2. Johnson GD, Medical Management of Migraine-Related Dizziness and Vertigo. *Laryngoscope* 1998;108 Supplement 85:1-28.

CHAPTER FIVE

Inner Ear Causes of Dizziness and Vertigo

Lloyd B. Minor, M.D.

Andelot Professor and Director

Department of Otolaryngology—Head and Neck Surgery
The Johns Hopkins University School of Medicine

Dr. Minor is the Andelot Professor and Chairman of the Department of Otolaryngology—Head and Neck Surgery at the Johns Hopkins University School of Medicine. He is an otologist and neurotologist with research interests in basic and clinical vestibular physiology. In 1998, Dr. Minor and his colleagues described a clinical syndrome of vertigo and balance disturbance caused by a dehiscence of bone overlying the superior semicircular canal. After making the discovery, he devised a surgical procedure to correct the abnormality. Other areas of interest include Ménière's disease and other inner ear disorders.

Disorders of the inner ear can cause symptoms and signs that are indicative of vestibular dysfunction. This chapter will review these symptoms and signs that can occur when there's a disturbance in the normal functional mechanisms of the inner ear. Specific disorders that can affect the inner ear will then be described. A diagram of the structures of the inner ear is shown in Figure 5-1.

But first let me tell you how fascinating the inner ear vestibular system is. The vestibular portion of the inner ear contains five endorgans to perceive different types of motion. They are exquisitely sensitive to head movement and transmit this information about head motion to the brain. The perceptual threshold for *angular acceleration* has been shown to be as low as $0.1°/second^2$. By way of comparison, a swivel chair accelerating at a constant rate of $0.1°/second^2$ would take 90 seconds to complete a single revolution.[1] Linear accelerations as small as a thousand times that of gravity can be detected by the Otolith organs. For example, an elevator mov-

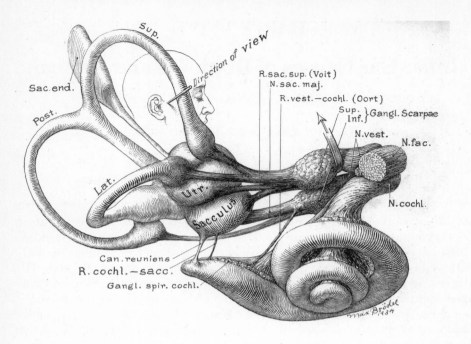

Figure 5-1: Drawings of the structures of the labyrinth. These structures include the utriculus (utr.), sacculus, anterior or superior semicircular canal (sup.), posterior semicircular canal (post.), and horizontal or lateral semicircular canal (lat.). The superior vesitbular nerve innervates the horizontal and superior canals and the utriculus. The inferior vestibular nerve innervates the posterior semicircular canal and the sacculus. The cell bodies for vestibular neurons are located in Scarpa's ganglion (Gangl. Scarpae).

ing at this acceleration would require almost 40 seconds to travel between floors.

Why is it important for the brain to receive exquisitely accurate information about head movement from the vestibular receptors? Many of the reflexes that are responsible for normal posture and balance and for maintaining steady visual fixation on objects during head movements depend upon information about the motion of the head coming from the labyrinth. While other sensory information (such as vision and the sense of touch) provides some information on motion, the signals from these other sensory systems are relatively slow and less accurate when compared to the information that comes from normal functioning vestibular receptors. Thus, symptoms and signs of vestibular dysfunction reflect abnormalities in motion perception (and in the information about motion received by the brain).

You'll recall that earlier in this book the Vestibulo-Ocular Reflex (VOR) was discussed. This is one of the most important reflexes controlled by the vestibular system. Remember that when it functions properly, this reflex enables us to maintain steady fixation on a stationary object while our head is moving.

Visual acuity during head movements is dependent upon the precisely calibrated function of the VOR. Deficits in vestibular function lead to impairments in the way the VOR attempts to compensate. Symptoms include *oscillopsia*, the apparent motion of objects that are known to be stationary during head movements. Acute changes in the level of neural activity arising from the labyrinth can result in vertigo, an illusion of motion. The symptom of *vertigo* is often accompanied by nystagmus, a rapid to-and-fro beating of the eyes caused by unequal activity between the two labyrinths.

Let's now explore inner ear causes of dizziness and vertigo.

Benign Paroxysmal Positional Vertigo (BPPV)

Benign paroxysmal positional vertigo (BPPV) is the most common cause of vertigo. It is characterized by rotational vertigo brought on when the head is rolled to the side, as when turning over in bed or when moving the head upward and to the side. Known causes of BPPV include head trauma, middle ear infection, migraine, viral labyrinthitis and prolonged bed rest. Half of occurrences have no clear precipitating event. BPPV occurs in children and in adults, although the incidence increases with age.

The vertigo typically begins after a short delay—up to 20 seconds after changing the position of the head—and continues for less than a minute. It is commonly provoked by the Dix-Hallpike maneuver (when a patient is moved rapidly from a sitting to a supine position, head turned to the side and shoulders hanging off the end of the examination table). Knowledge of the anatomy and physiology of the labyrinth has allowed practitioners to develop both a working theory for the cause of these symptoms as well as exercises to reverse them. Indeed, this sometimes crippling disease can often be completely cured in a single office visit.

BPPV most commonly affects the posterior semicircular canal. Calcium carbonate crystals, which are normally located in the membranous coverings overlying the Otolith organs, can become dislodged and accumulate in other areas of the labyrinth. The place where the crystals are likely to accumulate is in the most dependent location in the inner ear—the posterior semicircular canal. Motion of the head leads to movement of the crystals in the posterior canal. This results in an activation of the nerve fibers that innervate the posterior canal. The brain assumes that the information carried by the posterior canal nerve is caused by rotation of the head around the axis of the canal and creates a compensatory motion of the eyes—motion that is seen as nystagmus when a patient with BPPV is placed in the Dix-Hallpike position.

Current therapy for BPPV involves repositioning maneuvers that use gravity to move the crystals out of the affected semicircular canal and into the *vestibule* (the central chamber that contains the utricle and sacculus, the organs perceiving horizontal and vertical movements). These maneuvers are highly effective and surgical procedures are seldom needed.

Labyrinthitis and Vestibular Neuritis

Infectious and inflammatory processes can affect the inner ear. Hearing loss and vestibular disturbances can result if both the cochlea and the labyrinth are involved (*labyrinthitis*). Most such cases are assumed to have a viral etiology although it has proven difficult to isolate a specific virus in most cases. Steroids administered orally or in combination with steroid medication injected into the middle ear are often used in the treatment of acute episodes. Antiviral medications administered orally may also be beneficial.

When labyrinthitis is caused by a bacterial infection as in the case of a chronic middle ear and mastoid infection that spreads into the inner ear, prompt treatment with antibiotics and possible surgical removal of the infection is indicated. Bacterial labyrinthitis is encountered far less commonly than viral labyrinthitis.

Vestibular neuritis is characterized by the sudden onset of vertigo that lasts for days to weeks. Hearing is not impaired in cases of vestibular neuritis. Patients show clinical signs of loss of vestibular function in the affected ear and vestibular tests confirm this abnormality. The cause of vestibular neuritis remains an area of speculation and debate. Evidence in favor of an infection etiology comes from the observation of clusters of cases in a particular geographic location and at specific times of the year. A vascular etiology, however, is suggested by the observation that one division of the vestibular nerve is more often affected than the other. The vertigo, although initially quite severe, resolves over the course of days to weeks and vestibular tests performed weeks to months later often document recovery of function in the affected ear. There may be a higher incidence of BPPV in patients who have had a prior episode of vestibular neuritis.

Perilymphatic Fistula

The inner ear has distinct, fluid-filled compartments that are important for maintaining the functional capacity of the receptor cells responsible for hearing and balance. One of these fluids, *endolymph*, is high in potassium concentration. The other fluid, *perilymph*, is high in sodium concentration. These fluids are normally present in tightly constrained spaces. If the fluid can leak out into the middle ear it is called a *perilymphatic fistula*.

One situation in which the mechanism of perilymphatic fistula has been most convincingly established as a cause of hearing loss and vestibular disturbance involves an operation that opens the inner ear called stapedectomy. A *stapedectomy* is performed when the stapes bone (the third of the middle ear bones and smallest bone in the body) has become fixed to the surrounding bone by otosclerosis.

Otosclerosis is a hereditary condition causing bone remodeling around the inner ear. If the remodeling interferes with movement of the stapes bone that brings sound vibration into the inner ear, it can cause a *conductive hearing loss*. It is called a conductive hearing loss because sounds are heard better when conducted through bony parts of the head than through the ear itself. Replacement of the stuck (fixed) stapes with a prosthesis (an artificial replacement bone) is performed by making an opening into the inner ear. The opening is subsequently covered with the prosthesis and some surrounding material.

The procedure is highly effective at restoring normal hearing in most patients. In rare cases perilymph can leak into the middle ear leading to vertigo and hearing loss because loss of perilymph disturbs the function of the receptor cells in the inner ear. Prompt closure of the leakage can lead to restoration of hearing and balance function. Perilymphatic fistula can also occur following head trauma, barotrauma and explosive blasts near the ear.

There is controversy surrounding the possible occurrence of a perilymphatic fistula without a specific event or injury prior to the onset of symptoms. The debate concerning such 'idiopathic' perilymphatic fistulas is made more complicated because surgical exploration in many cases has failed to reveal a fistula or leakage of fluid into the middle ear. The surgical treatment in such cases has involved placement of soft tissue graft to seal the possible fistula in the most likely locations. These locations are around the oval and round windows.

Superior Canal Dehiscence Syndrome

A syndrome of vertigo induced by loud noises or by changes in middle ear or inner ear pressures has recently been recognized in patients with a defect in the superior semicircular canal. These patients may also experience chronic dysequilibrium. There are normally only two movable windows in the inner ear and rest of the inner ear is surrounded by hard bone. Sound normally enters the inner ear through movements of the stapes bone into the oval window. The sound travels through the cochlea and exits at the round window which contains a thin flexible membrane.

All of the semicircular canals are encased in solid bone. The uppermost canal, the superior canal, and the one closest to the brain cavity, can sometimes be eroded by the brain cavity leaving an opening (dehiscence) in the bone covered by the membranes that protect the brain. The dehiscence creates a third mobile window into the inner ear thereby allowing the superior canal to respond to sound or changes in pressure in the ear or head. Patients with this syndrome are often observed to have eye movements evoked by loud noises or by pressure changes. Some of the activities that can cause these pressure changes include coughing, straining, nose blowing and pushing on the outer ear.

Some of the symptoms experienced by patients with this syndrome may at first seem bizarre. Patients may experience a bobbing of their vision in association with their pulse or they may complain that they "hear" their eye movements. All of these symptoms can be understood in terms of the effects of the dehiscence on the physiology of the inner ear.

Specific findings on clinical examination and the results of diagnostic tests are used to determine if a patient has superior canal dehiscence syndrome. The eye movements that are evoked by the sound or pressure stimuli align with the plane of the affected superior canal. These eye movements can be observed by the clinician and can be recorded with special video techniques. Another test that is useful in the diagnosis of this syndrome involves the use of loud tones to cause a reflex response in the neck muscles. This response is recorded with electrodes on the skin overlying the muscles. These *vestibular evoked myogenic potentials* or VEMP (a test that involves use of sounds in the ear that cause an inner ear reflex response) most likely arise from the sacculus, one of the vestibular endorgans in the inner ear. Patients with superior canal dehiscence syndrome have an abnormally low threshold for this response arising from the affected ear. The opening in the bone overlying the superior canal can be revealed by a CT scan of the temporal bone. The scan needs to be performed with special resolution and display techniques so as not to miss a layer of bone that is intact but thin.

Establishing an accurate diagnosis is important because the symptoms experienced by these patients can be seen, in varying combinations, with other disorders affecting the inner ear or the nervous system. Some patients with superior canal dehiscence syndrome had previously been suspected to have a perilymphatic fistula and had undergone middle ear surgery for a fistula without any improvement in symptoms. Once the diagnosis of superior canal dehiscence syndrome is established, many patients are able to control their symptoms by avoiding the sounds or activities that cause vestibular disturbances. A surgical procedure to repair the dehiscence has been used with success in patients for whom the symptoms were debilitating.

Some patients may have primarily hearing symptoms such as conductive hearing loss or distortion. The hearing loss may be confused with otosclerosis. Auditory and vestibular screening tests such as acoustic reflex responses and VEMPs are useful in making the distinction between these causes of conductive hearing loss. When due to a problem with the bones in the middle ear, the responses on these tests will be absent. When due to superior canal dehiscence, the responses are still present and the VEMP is stronger than normal.

Ménière's Disease

Patients with Ménière's disease experience episodes of vertigo, fluctuating hearing loss, tinnitus and aural fullness (a painful pressure sensation in the ear). This disorder most commonly affects only one ear although during the course of the disease both ears may ultimately be affected in some people. The attacks of vertigo are often preceded by an increase in tinnitus or aural fullness or by a decline in hearing in the affected ear. Patients often experience transient improvement in hearing immediately following an episode of vertigo.

An attack of vertigo in Ménière's disease typically lasts from 20 minutes to three to four hours. The vertigo involves a strong spinning sensation and is usually accompanied by nausea or vomiting. Patients may have unsteadiness, disequilibrium and fatigue that last for several hours after the spinning stops. Less commonly, patients may have episodes that involve a sudden loss of balance as the manifestation of an attack of Ménière's disease. Patients often describe these spells as a feeling that the floor moves out from underneath them. Falls can occur unless there's a stationary object nearby for patients to stabilize their balance. These sudden "drop attacks" are thought to be due to the effects of Ménière's disease on the Otolith organs.

Ménière's disease is thought to be caused by an over-production or over-accumulation of endolymph (one of the inner ear fluids). The reason this occurs is not clear in most instances. The disorder afflicts over 600,000 Americans. For many of them, the unpredictable episodes of vertigo are the most debilitating symptom.

Episodes of vertigo in Ménière's disease can often be controlled with a low sodium diet and diuretics (medications that reduce fluid in the inner ear). Steroid medications and vestibular suppressants may also be beneficial during times when the vertigo is particularly severe.

A number of treatments have been used when the episodes of vertigo are not controlled by these medical measures. Surgical procedures to decompress the *endolymphatic sac* (located in the inner ear where endolymph accumulates) have been used. The vestibular nerve can be cut and thereby eliminate the signals that are responsible for triggering an episode of vertigo.

Over the past decade, attention has been focused at many centers on the development of protocols for the injection of gentamicin in the middle ear to control vertigo. Gentamicin is toxic to the receptor cells in the vestibular system. A single injection of gentamicin into the middle ear is typically sufficient to cause the reduction in vestibular function that is required to control vertigo. The risk of hearing loss caused by such a treatment is low.

Acoustic Neuroma

Tumors arising along the nerves that course from the inner ear to the brain can cause disturbances of hearing and balance. These tumors are commonly referred to as *acoustic neuromas* although the more accurate term used to describe them is *vestibular schwannomas*. They typically arise from the vestibular nerves that carry information about head movement from the labyrinth to the brain. The tumors begin as abnormal growths of the schwann cells (which provide the lining around the nerve fibers traveling in the vestibular nerves). These tumors are not cancers in that they don't metastasize (spread) to lymph nodes. However, by virtue of their location, they can cause disturbances of hearing and balance. If they grow to a large size, then they can compress the brainstem and result in serious neurological dysfunction.

Even though the tumors arise from the vestibular nerves, the presenting symptoms are usually abnormalities of hearing such as tinnitus (ringing in the ear) and hearing loss in the affected ear. Vertigo and other complaints related specifically to balance are relatively uncommon. Tests of vestibular function such as the caloric test will often reveal a weakness of function in the affected ear. Many patients experience no symptoms related to the diminished vestibular function. This is because these tumors grow slowly and the brain has a remarkable capacity to adapt to changes in vestibular function in one ear that occur over the course of weeks and months. Hearing loss, tinnitus and distorted sounds in the affected ear occur as a consequence of the tumor pushing against, and resulting in dysfunction of the hearing nerve. These hearing-related symptoms are most commonly the ones which lead patients to seek medical attention.

Patients with a vestibular schwannoma may experience vertigo. The most accurate method for identification of these tumors is with a magnetic resonance imaging (MRI) scan with the intravenous administration of gadolinium (a contrast agent that makes the tumors highly visible). Other indications for obtaining an MRI scan to evaluate for a vestibular neuroma can include hearing loss that is worse in one ear than the other and auditory symptoms such as tinnitus that localize to one ear.

Otosclerosis

Otosclerosis is the most common disorder of the middle ear bones not resulting from an infectious process. The underlying pathology is an abnormality of the footplate of the stapes bone, the third of the three bones in the middle ear. Motion of this stapes bone is normally responsible for the transmission of sound into the inner ear. Patients develop a conductive hearing loss when the footplate of the stapes becomes fixed due to otosclerosis. The intensity of sound transmitted through the air is diminished although sound transmitted directly through the bone of the skull is heard at normal threshold. Two-thirds of patients affected with otosclerosis are women. The hearing loss usually begins in the teens or 20s and may be accelerated during pregnancy. A hearing aid can be beneficial. Alternatively, an operation to replace the stapes bone leads to improvement in hearing in the majority of cases.

It has been suggested that inner ear otosclerosis may be a cause of symptoms of vertigo, tinnitus and fluctuating hearing loss in some patients, although controversy exists as to whether it can cause disturbances of vestibular function. Patients with Ménière's disease and otosclerosis have been identified but it's not clear whether there's a causal relationship between these two disorders or whether their concurrent existence in a patient is coincidence.

Loss of Vestibular Function due to *Ototoxic* Drugs

Treatment of infections with intravenous of aminoglycoside antibiotics can result in damage to the vestibular receptor cells in the inner ear. Gentamicin is the most commonly used aminoglycoside antibiotic in the U.S. Damage to vestibular function as a consequence of gentamicin administration can occur without loss of hearing and may result even when levels of the antibiotic in the blood are maintained within the therapeutic range. Vestibular toxicity is more likely when the administration of gentamicin is continued for periods longer than 10 days.

Patients who develop vestibular injury from gentamicin usually do not experience vertigo. The reason for the lack of vertigo is that the decline in vestibular function is occurring in both ears at relatively the same rate. Vertigo as a symptom results when there is an imbalance in vestibular activity between the two sides. Oscillopsia with head movements is a common symptom associated with development of gentamicin-induced vestibular toxicity. Patients have difficulty reading and maintaining good visual acuity with head movements. They may also have an unstable gait and difficulty maintaining their balance with their eyes closed. Discontinuation of the antibiotic at the time that symptoms and signs of vestibular injury first begin may reduce the severity of the inner ear damage.

Vertigo caused by Neurological Disorders

Vertigo is a symptom caused by a disturbance in function somewhere along the vestibular pathways. In addition to inner ear disorders we have discussed, pathologies affecting the brainstem or cerebellum can also result in vertigo. It's important that these central nervous system disorders be distinguished from inner ear abnormalities. Strokes affecting the brainstem or cerebellum can lead to vertigo. In the case of brainstem involvement, the vertigo will be accompanied by other neurological signs and symptoms that will point to the cause. A stroke in the cerebellum can, however, result in vertigo and in vestibular signs that mimic an inner ear disorder. The primary distinguishing feature is that patients with an acute stroke affecting the cerebellum typically cannot stand or walk whereas patients with vertigo due to an inner ear abnormality can stand and walk although they are likely to be unsteady. Suspicion must be maintained in patients who present the acute onset of vertigo and gait abnormalities. Imaging of the brain provides an accurate method for detection of an infarction or hemorrhage of the cerebellum. In the case of a hemorrhage, prompt removal of the blood clot is required in order to prevent more extensive neurological damage.

References

1. Fuchs AF. Excitable cells and neurophysiology. In Textbook of Physiology, vol 1, Fuchs AF et al, ed. Philidelphia: W B Saunders Co., 1989: 587.

CHAPTER SIX

Benign Paroxysmal Positional Vertigo (BPPV)

Lorne Parnes MD, FRCSC
Professor, Departments of Otolaryngology and Clinical Neurological
Sciences, University of Western Ontario, London, Canada

Lorne Parnes, MD, is Professor and Chair of the Department of Otolaryngology and Professor of Clinical Neurological Sciences at the University if Western Ontario in London, Canada where he also serves as Chief of Otolaryngology at both the London Health Sciences Centre and St. Joseph's Health Centre. He has published extensively and lectured internationally about the causes, mechanisms and various treatments of benign paroxysmal positional vertigo (BPPV). He pioneered the posterior semicircular canal occlusion procedure which is currently the surgical procedure of choice for intractable BPPV. Dr. Parnes is also renowned for his work on direct drug delivery implementation in the treatment of various other inner ear diseases.

Introduction

For some, a session with the bed spins is a terrifying event that might occur during an alcoholic binge. Imagine though that while perfectly sober, each time you lay down, turn over in bed or look up, you launch into such a spin. This is the essence of benign paroxysmal positional vertigo (BPPV). Fortunately, unlike the alcohol related bed spin, the BPPV spin (technically known as *vertigo*) lasts but for a few seconds and rarely results in vomiting. Unfortunately, it can occur with each and every such head movement for weeks to months (and rarely years) on end.

Of all of the inner ear disorders that can cause dizziness/vertigo, benign paroxysmal positional vertigo (BPPV) is by far the most common, occurring in about one in five patients seen in dizziness clinics. It is a condition that is usually easily diagnosed and, even more importantly, readily treated with a simple office-based procedure. Dr. Robert Barany, the Austrian neurologist/otologist who won the Nobel Prize in Physiology/ Medicine in 1914 for his work on the physiology and pathology of the vestibular (balance) apparatus, first described the condition in 1921. He gave the following account from one of his patients:

"The attacks only appeared when she lay on her right side. When she did this, there appeared a strong rotatory nystagmus to the right. The attack lasted about thirty seconds and was accompanied by violent vertigo and nausea. If, immediately after the cessation of these symptoms, the head was again turned to the right, no attack occurred, and in order to evoke a new attack in this way, the patient had to lie for some time on her back or on her left side."

Since this initial description, there have been major advances in the understanding of this common condition. In this chapter, I will review the normal vestibular physiology as it relates to BPPV, discuss the causes and mechanisms of BPPV, and then go on to discuss diagnostic tests, office-based management, and finally, surgical management.

Anatomy and Physiology

The vestibular system monitors the body's motion and position in space by detecting rotational and linear movements of the head. In a previous chapter, you learned that it is the three semicircular canals that detect rotational movements, technically referred to as *angular acceleration*. These canals are positioned at near right angles to each other so as to detect rotation in any plane in space. Each canal contains a membranous tube filled with a fluid called *endolymph*, which is in turn surrounded and cushioned by a second fluid called *perilymph*. Each has a swelling at one end of the canal termed the *ampulla*. The ampulla contains the gelatine-like membrane called the *cupula*, in which are embedded the hair cells. The cupula, which is "floating" in the endolymph fluid, is induced to move in one direction or the other depending on which way the head turns. This in turn stimulates the hair cells. The variation of the signals from the hair cells induces variations in the impulses in the balance nerves which, under normal circumstances, are interpreted by the brain as a head movement. However in the condition BPPV, the cupula is forced to move by an unnatural mechanism that occurs with the head at rest. The resulting abnormal nerve impulse tricks the brain into thinking that the head and body are moving when in fact they are not. The end result is an illusion that the environment is spinning. Think of the time in your childhood when you used to spin yourself around and around and then abruptly come to a stop. Remember how you lost your balance while it felt like the world kept on spinning, and then after a few seconds the spinning would slowly fade away. It is this exact same mechanism that results, and the same feeling that ensues, in BPPV.

Technical Terminology

Ampullofugal refers to movement 'away' from the ampulla, whereas *ampullopetal* refers to movement 'toward' the ampulla. In the superior and posterior semicircular canals, ampullofugal movement of the cupula excites and ampullopetal deflection inhibits the hair cells and nerves. The converse is true for the lateral semicircular canal.

Nystagmus refers to the repeated and rhythmical oscillation of the eyes. Abnormal nerve impulses from the semicircular canals most commonly cause *jerk nystagmus*, characterized by a slow phase (slow, accelerating movement in one direction) followed by a fast phase (rapid return to the original position). The direction of the nystagmus is named after the direction of the fast phase. Nystagmus can be horizontal, vertical, oblique, rotatory, or any combination thereof. *Geotropic nystagmus* refers to nystagmus beating toward the ground, whereas apo-*ageotropic nystagmus* refers to nystagmus beating away from the ground.

Canalithiasis (canal, meaning tube & lithiasis, meaning *stones*) describes the concept that there is free-floating debris within the semicircular canal endolymph. The concept was first described in 1979 by Dr. Joseph McClure and colleagues in London, Ontario, and the phenomenon was first confirmed by me during surgery in 1992. *Cupulolithiasis* alludes to the concept that debris (*stones*) is stuck to the cupula of the semicircular canal. This term was coined by Dr. Harold Schuknecht of Boston, in 1969.

Otoconia, sometimes referred to as "ear rocks", are normal occurring microscopic calcium matrix crystals that are embedded in the membrane of the otolith receptors. These are the receptors that are responsible for detecting linear forces or movements, one example of which is gravity. In most cases, displaced otoconia are the "stones", "debris" or "particles" that are responsible for both cupulolithiasis and canalithiasis. I have actually removed the particles from a posterior canal in a patient undergoing surgery for severe BPPV (see later in chapter). Ultra-high power microscopic analysis (scanning electron microscopy) demonstrated that, at least in this one patient, the particles were indeed otoconia. Through various mechanisms, these otoconia would have to become dislodged from the utricular otolithic membrane in which they are normally imbedded, leaving them floating freely in the endolymph. Through naturally occurring head movements, these "stones" migrate into one of the semicircular canals (canalithiasis) or become adherent to one of the cupulae (cupulolithiasis) to cause the BPPV.

Mechanism

BPPV can be caused by either canalithiasis or cupulolithiasis, and each of these mechanisms can theoretically affect any of the three semicircular canals.

Posterior (Inferior) Canal BPPV

The vast majority of all BPPV cases arise in the posterior semicircular canal. As well, the underlying mechanism causing the majority of posterior canal BPPV is thought to be *canalithiasis*. This is because free-floating endolymph debris gets pulled down into the posterior canal since it is the most gravity dependent part of the inner ear balance organ whether a person is either standing or lying flat on their back. Once debris enters the posterior canal, the cupular barrier at the shorter, more dependent end of the canal blocks exit of the debris. Therefore, the debris becomes 'trapped' and can only exit at the non-ampullated end (the *common crus*) which under normal conditions would necessitate the particles moving upward, away from gravity.

Dr. John Epley at the Portland (Oregon) Otologic Clinic, has been one of the most influential physicians to elaborate on the mechanism underlying, and the treatment of, BPPV. Dr. Epley has explained that canalithiasis causes nystagmus in the posterior semicircular canal when particles (debris) accumulate to a "critical mass" in the dependent portion of the canal. When the orientation of the semicircular canal is modified in the plane of gravity, such as what happens when an affected person looks up or rolls over in bed, the canalith mass moves to a more dependent position. The hydrodynamic drag of the mass must overcome the resistance of the endolymph in the semicircular canal and the elasticity of the cupular barrier in order to deflect (move) the cupula. The time taken for this to occur plus the original inertia of the particles accounts for the fact there is usually a delayed response of a few seconds between the movement of the head and the onset of the vertigo. To test for BPPV of the posterior semicircular canal we use the Dix-Hallpike maneuver, and this will be described in more detail later in the chapter.

Lateral (Horizontal) Canal BPPV

Although BPPV most commonly arises in the posterior semicircular canal, it has been reported that as many as 30 percent of BPPV cases may be of the horizontal canal variant. In my dizziness clinic, the horizontal canal variant accounts for less than 5 percent of cases of positional vertigo. However, these findings may be biased by the long wait for an assessment in my clinic (greater than five months), as it has also been my experience that lateral canal BPPV resolves much quicker than posterior canal BPPV. These observations are understandable when one considers the orientations of the canals. The posterior canal hangs down and has its cupular barrier at its shorter, more dependent end. Any debris entering the canal essentially becomes trapped within it. The lateral canal slopes up and has its cupular barrier at the upper end. Therefore free-floating debris in the lateral canal would tend to float back out into the utricle just with natural head movements. Just like in the posterior canal, both cupulolithiasis and canalithiasis are implicated as the underlying mechanism. Since it is much easier to treat, it is fortunate that the latter mechanism is much more common, as it is in posterior canal BPPV.

Lateral canal BPPV can be induced during the office based treatment for posterior canal BPPV (see later in chapter). As long as it recognized by the treating clinician, it should be easy to fix by a simple alteration of the treatment.

Superior (Anterior) Canal BPPV

Superior canal BPPV is a very, very rare condition which, like the lateral canal variant, is usually self-limited. I have personally not seen this variant in my own clinic, but because it is so rare and self limited, I may have overlooked it on occasion.

Prevalence

As mentioned previously, BPPV is the most common disorder that affects the balance part of the inner ear. Several reports have suggested a higher incidence in women, but in younger patients, and those with BPPV arising from head trauma, the incidence is equal between men and women. The age of onset is most commonly during the fifth to seventh decades of life. The elderly also seem to be at an increased risk, and one study of an elderly population undergoing geriatric assessment for non-balance-related complaints found that 9 percent had unrecognized BPPV. BPPV most often involves a single semicircular canal, usually posterior, but may involve both posterior and lateral canals in the same inner ear. Posterior canal BPPV may convert to lateral canal BPPV following repositioning maneuvers (see later in chapter for discussion). Head trauma, usually from a fall or motor vehicle accident, is the most common cause of BPPV in younger people. It is also the most common situation where we would find BPPV affecting both inner ears simultaneously.

Causes

In most cases, BPPV is found in isolation and as such, it is termed *primary* or *idiopathic* BPPV. This type accounts for about 50-70 percent of cases. The most common cause of *secondary* BPPV is *head trauma*, representing 7-17% of all BPPV cases. The blow to the head would cause the release of numerous otoconia into the endolymph, which likely explains why many of these patients suffer from bilateral BPPV. A viral inner ear infection is the next most common known cause, and it has been implicated in up to 15% of BPPV cases. In these cases of viral infections, there would be an initial period with several days of severe, constant vertigo. This would gradually resolve and sometime later, anywhere from a few days to a few weeks, change into the more positional type of vertigo that we see in BPPV.

Ménière's disease has also been shown to be associated with BPPV. As discussed in Chapter 7, people with Ménière's disease have more intense, longer-lasting (30 minutes-24 hours) but less frequent vertigo spells than those with BPPV. The spells are not brought on by positional change, and unlike in BPPV, there are also symptoms affecting the organ of hearing in the inner ear including a fluctuating hearing loss and tinnitus (head noises). If hearing loss and/or tinnitus accompanies your vertigo spells, then it cannot be due to BPPV alone. The exact mechanism that results in the Ménière's disease and BPPV association is not well understood. One theory is that of Ménière's disease induced mechanical or biochemical damage to the macula of the utricle, with subsequent release of the otoconia into the endolymph.

Recently, *migraine headaches* have been found to be closely associated with BPPV. Since migraine in itself is so much more common among females, this may help explain the higher rate of BPPV among females in the general population. Migraines are thought to result from spasm and then dilation of the blood vessels going to the scalp and brain. It has been suggested that spasm of the inner ear arteries, which are branches of the arteries supplying the base of the brain, might lead to the damage of the otolith receptors which in turn results in release of the otoconia. It would also help to explain the high recurrence rate of BPPV in patients with migraine.

Secondary BPPV has also been described after inner ear surgery, most commonly stapedectomy, which is an operation done to correct hearing loss. The mechanism in this situation is thought to be mechanical damage to the otolith receptor, once again leading to the release of otoconia.

Diagnosis

History

People with BPPV have sudden, severe attacks of either horizontal or vertical vertigo, or a combination of both. When the attacks occur while lying down, many will say that it feels like they are falling or that the foot of the bed is coming up over their head. The attacks are almost always brought on by certain head positions and movements. The most common movements include rolling in bed, extending the neck to look up, and bending forward. Patients can often identify the affected ear by identifying the direction of movement which precipitates the majority of the attacks (e.g. if rolling in bed to the right, but not the left, precipitates the dizziness, it would indicate right ear involvement). I often ask patients this question to help me localize the side (ear) to test first. While the vast majority of patients describe feeling an intense spinning sensation, others experience more of a floating sensation. Some become severely frightened, while others become extremely nauseated, but rarely to the point of vomiting. These latter patients will go to great lengths to avoid those positions that bring on the vertigo. I've had some patients that have avoided the movements that bring on the vertigo for so long, that they weren't even aware of the fact that the disease had resolved on its own, as it usually does over time. They are often surprised (and delighted) when their test for BPPV comes up negative. Although the attacks of vertigo typically last less than 30 seconds, some patients greatly overestimate the duration of their "attacks," mostly because the fear response makes the attacks feel longer than they actually are. The majority of patients will experience several attacks per day.

In addition to vertigo, many patients complain of lightheadedness, nausea, imbalance, and in severe cases, sensitivity to all directions of head movement. Some patients are also extremely anxious for two other reasons. Some fear that the symptoms may represent some kind of sinister underlying disorder such as a brain tumour, while for others the symptoms are just too unsettling.

As the name implies, BPPV is most often a benign condition. However in certain situations it may become dangerous. For example, a painter looking up from the top of a ladder may suddenly become vertiginous and lose his or her balance, risking a bad fall. The same would hold true for underwater divers who might get very disoriented from acute vertigo. Heavy machinery operators should use great caution especially if their job involves significant head movement. Most people feel safe to drive their car so long as they're careful not to tip their head back when checking their blind spot.

Aside from the danger it may pose, for some, the disease can greatly impact their lives. Work performance may be affected, which of course depends on the activities of the job. For those afraid to lie down or turn on the affected side in bed, sleep can be greatly disturbed, which in itself can be very disabling. I've had a few patients complain about the disease's impact on their sexual activities. Mostly though, this disorder causes inconvenience in normal day to day activities. Shopping, cleaning, gardening, hair washing, putting in eye drops, reaching for an item on a high shelf, shaving, even drinking or just nodding yes are all activities that move the head vertically and potentially stimulate the inner ear in this disorder.

Prior to the development of effective treatments, the natural history of this condition was well-documented. Basically, there were three variants of primary BPPV. The most common form was "self-limited" BPPV that occurred suddenly, resolved in weeks to months, and did not recur. In the "recurrent" form, patients had multiple recurrent episodes of positional vertigo lasting weeks or months at a time interspersed with symptom-free periods lasting weeks to months or even years at a time. In the "permanent" form, the positional vertigo persisted without remission for greater than 1 year.

Although 50-70 percent of BPPV is *idiopathic* (no identifiable cause), possible secondary causes for BPPV should be identified. As mentioned previously, these include head trauma, viral inner ear infections, Ménière's disease, migraine headaches, and inner ear surgery. Your doctor should question you about symptoms of other inner ear or brain disorders, as on the rare occasion some of these may mimic BPPV.

Physical Examination

After taking a detailed history, the diagnosis of BPPV may be quite obvious. Nevertheless, your doctor will likely want to perform a neurotologic examination. This would include an examination of the ears, which might also include a hearing test. An examination of the cranial nerves is also important, and since the inner ear has direct connections with the eye muscles, detailed attention will be given to your eye movements looking specifically for nystagmus, which is an unusual rhythmic movement of the eyes.

Other areas to assess might include balance, co-ordination, posture and gait.

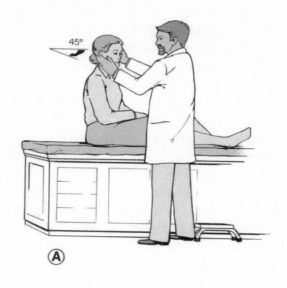

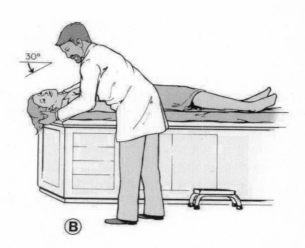

Figure 6-1:Dix–Hallpike Maneuver (right ear). In this case with the right side being tested, in position B your examiner should expect to see a fast-phase counter-clockwise nystagmus. To complete the maneuver, you will be returned to the seated position (A) and your eyes will be observed for reversal nystagmus—in this case a fast-phase clockwise nystagmus.

The Dix-Hallpike maneuver (Figure 6-1), first described in 1952, is the confirmatory test for "posterior canal" BPPV. To do this test, the patient is seated lengthwise on an examination table and positioned such that when laid back, their head will extend back over the edge of the table. Each inner ear is tested independent from the other. Initially the head is turned 45° toward the ear being tested and the patient is quickly lowered into the supine position with the head extending below the level of the table. The patient's head is held in this position and the examiner observes the eyes for a very specific nystagmus. Some people become quite anxious during this part of test, and have a tendency to close their eyes. However, it is most important for them to relax and try to keep their eyes open. Sometimes the examiner must go so far as to forcefully open the eyelids.

Typically the nystagmus starts anywhere from one to five seconds after lowering the head. It will increase in intensity, plateau and then decrease in intensity over a duration of about 15 -25 seconds. With the eyes in the mid (neutral) position, the nystagmus has a slight vertical component, the fast phase of which is up-beating. Of more clinical importance is the stronger rotational component, the fast phase of which has the superior pole of the eye beating toward the affected (dependent) ear. Clinicians will often refer to this as a clockwise nystagmus as seen in a positive test on the left side, or a counter-clockwise nystagmus arising from a positive test on the right. When the patient is brought back up to the sitting position, the nystagmus will reverse direction. That is, a clockwise response with the left ear down will reverse to a counter-clockwise response after returning to the sitting position, and vice versa for the right ear. Also, with a positive response, the patient will feel vertiginous, the intensity of which parallels the intensity of the nystagmus. Many patients are amazed by the fact that I can tell them when their vertigo starts and stops during this test simply by looking at their eyes. If the test is repeated over and over, the nystagmus and vertigo will grow weaker each time until it is gone. This is described as test fatigue. I would like to re-emphasize that the two posterior canals are tested independently, the right with the head turned right and the left with the head turned left.

Testing for "lateral canal" BPPV is done by laying the patient supine and then quickly turning the patient's head (and body if necessary) laterally toward the side being tested. In the majority of cases, a purely horizontal geotropic nystagmus occurs (fast component toward the lowermost ear) but some may show an apo-geotropic (fast component toward the uppermost ear) nystagmus. Compared to the vertical-torsional nystagmus of posterior canal BPPV, this horizontal nystagmus has a shorter latency, stronger intensity and longer duration when maintaining the test position, and it is less prone to fatigue. It also causes a more intense sensation of vertigo with patients who are more likely to vomit during positional testing. Both sides are tested and the direction of nystagmus coupled with the direction of roll causing the stronger nystagmus often identifies the affected side and the mechanism (cupulolithiasis or canalithiasis). Just like in posterior canal BPPV, it is important for your clinician to identify the side and mechanism so that they can direct their treatment accordingly.

Overall, the history and eye-findings during positional testing are by far the most valuable pieces of information for diagnosing BPPV. Once in awhile, a patient with a classic BPPV history shows no response during the Dix-Hallpike (for posterior canal) or lateral head turn (for lateral canal) testing. Not uncommonly if such a patient returned on another day, a repeat positional test might prove to be positive. Conversely, if I see a patient with a history of recurring BPPV who has not had any recent spells, I wouldn't expect to see any abnormalities during the examination. I ask these patients to call my office if and when their symptoms recur so that I can examine them when their symptoms are actively present.

Additional testing is not normally required to make, or support, the diagnosis. Since electronystagmography (ENG) does not record the rotational eye movements that dominate the nystagmus of BPPV, it adds very little information. More recently, infrared videography has allowed for direct eye observation during the testing maneuvers. This can help the examiner to observe the eye movements without having to bend over. Rotational chair testing and posturography have no role to play in this disorder. Brain imaging with CT scan or MRI is unnecessary unless there are atypical or unusual features of the assessment, or surgery is being considered.

Subjective vs. Objective BPPV

A certain subset of patients may not demonstrate any nystagmus during the Dix-Hallpike maneuver, but may still experience the typical time course of vertigo during the test. This has been termed "subjective" BPPV. There are various theories as to why this might occur, but more importantly, several studies have found repositioning maneuvers (discussed in next section) to be almost as highly effective in this group of patients as it is in the more typical (objective) group.

Other Conditions Need to be Excluded (Differential Diagnosis)

There are very few conditions that can even remotely resemble BPPV. In Ménière's disease, the vertigo spells are not provoked by position change, and they last much longer (30 minutes to several hours). Furthermore, there is accompanying tinnitus and hearing loss. The vertigo in viral *labyrinthitis/vestibular neuronitis* usually persists for days. The vertigo may be aggravated by head movements in any direction, and this needs to be carefully extracted from the history so as to not confuse it with specific position change evoked vertigo. As well, the Dix-Hallpike test should not induce the burst of nystagmus seen in BPPV. Very rarely, brain tumors can mimic BPPV, but there have been no reports in the literature in which a tumor has perfectly replicated all of the features seen in a positive Dix-Hallpike maneuver. As mentioned previously, BPPV can be secondary, so as to occur concurrently with, or subsequent to, other inner ear or CNS disorders.

Table 6-1: Quick Fact Table

Diagnosis of BPPV
History

-Spinning dizziness
  -Lasts less than 30 seconds
  -brought on by certain head movements

Dix-Hallpike Maneuver for Posterior Canal BPPV

-Short delay before the onset of nystagmus and vertigo
  -Limited duration of response (15-30 seconds)
  -Torsional nystagmus that is ear specific
  -Reversal of nystagmus upon sitting
  -Fades with repeated testing

Lateral Head Turns for Horizontal Canal BPPV
-Geotropic nystagmus (canalithiasis)   -Apo-geotropic nystagmus (cupulolithiasis)
Subjective BPPV
-Vertigo during Dix-Hallpike test   -No nystagmus seen
-Repositioning maneuvers still effective

Non-Surgical Management

Traditionally, patients were instructed to avoid positions which induced the vertigo. Medications have been found to be ineffective in preventing or stopping the vertigo. Alternative treatments such as vitamins, naturopathy and holistic medications have not been well studied in the medical literature.

With the progressive understanding of its underlying mechanism, the management of BPPV has changed dramatically in the past 20 years. BPPV is usually self-limited and the majority of cases resolve over several months. As the theories of cupulolithiasis and canalithiasis emerged, several non-invasive techniques were developed to hasten the recovery.

Vestibular Habituation Therapy

In 1980, when BPPV was still felt to result from cupulolithiasis in most cases, Brandt and Daroff introduced a specific series of positional movements/exercises. They felt that the exercises caused the mechanical loosening and dispersion of otolithic debris from the cupula. The set of exercises were to be done every three hours during the day until two days after the positional vertigo had resolved. Others believed that these exercises worked by training the brain to "ignore" the abnormal nerve impulses from the diseased inner ear. In all likelihood, these exercises worked in a similar (although not as effective) fashion as particle repositioning, to be discussed next. Although vestibular habituation has been shown to be more effective than no treatment, the exercises are time-consuming and poorly tolerated by some patients, especially the obese and the elderly.

Liberatory Maneuver

In 1988, the French physiotherapist Dr. Alain Semont first described the *liberatory maneuver* based on the theory of cupulolithiasis being the underlying mechanism of BPPV. Dr. Semont believed that this series of rapid changes of head position freed deposits that were attached to the cupula. The maneuver begins with the patient in the sitting position and head turned away from the affected side (see Figure 6-2). The patient is then quickly put into the side-lying position, toward the affected side, with the patient's head turned upward. After approximately five minutes, the patient is quickly moved back through the sitting position to the opposite side-lying position with their head now facing downward. To be effective, this step must be done rapidly! The patient remains in this second position for 5-10 minutes before slowly being brought back to the sitting position.

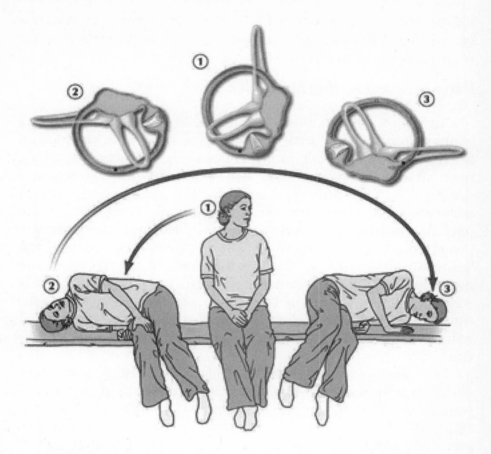

Figure 6-2: Liberatory Maneuver of Semont (right ear). The top panel shows the effect of the maneuver on the labyrinth as viewed from the front and the induced movement of the particles (black dots). This maneuver relies on inertia, so that the transition from position 2 to 3 must be made very quickly.

Several dizzy clinics around the world have reported response rates of up to 93 percent with recurrence rates of up to 29 percent. There has been no difference in efficacy shown between the *liberatory maneuver* and *particle repositioning maneuver*, to be discussed next. In my opinion, the liberatory maneuver is very effective, but is difficult to perform in elderly, frail or obese patients, which is why I prefer the particle repositioning maneuver.

Particle Repositioning Maneuver

Although he had been teaching his technique for many years prior, it wasn't until 1992 that Dr. John Epley published his first report on the *canalith repositioning procedure* (CRP), now simply known as the Epley maneuver. His original description of the procedure included the use of pre-treatment sedative medication and mechanical skull vibration as the patient's head was moved sequentially through five separate positions. Dr. Epley proposed that the procedure induced the "canalithis" to move under the influence of gravity from the posterior semicircular canal back into the utricle, which is where they came from in the first place. Skull vibration was thought to help "jiggle" the particles through the fluid. I believe that most clinicians today use a modified version of the CRP.

One modified CRP is the particle repositioning maneuver (PRM) which is a three-position maneuver that eliminates the routine use of sedation and skull vibration, although both are sometimes used in certain situations. So long as they understand the inner ear anatomy and the mechanism that underlies BPPV, appropriately trained health professionals, including family doctors and physiotherapists, should be able to successfully carry out the PRM in most straight forward cases. Unusual cases or those that do not respond to the conventional treatment should be referred to a specialized "dizzy" clinic. I would strongly advise against trying to do these maneuvers at home without supervision for two reasons. First, it is difficult for lay people to understand the 3-dimensional anatomy of the inner ear which is of the utmost importance when performing these maneuvers. Second, the correct diagnosis needs to be made with specific respect to the side of involvement, the canal involved and the mechanism (canal- vs. cupulo-lithiasis). To sort this out, it is important to have a trained person observe your eyes during the testing.

In the following sequence, I will outline the important steps of the PRM: (see Figure 6-3, page 144).

1. You are placed in a sitting position, lengthwise on an examination table (position A);

2. You'll be asked to turn your head 45 degrees to the side being tested;

3. You'll move your head to the head-hanging (Dix-Hallpike) position of the test ear (position B);

4. Your eyes will be observed for nystagmus (we call this the primary stage nystagmus);

5. You'll maintain this position for 1-2 minutes;

6. You'll be asked to turn your head 90 degrees to the opposite side while keeping the neck in full extension (position C);

7. You'll continue to roll another 90 degrees until your head is diagonally opposite to the first Dix-Hallpike position D (the change from position B, through C, into D, should take no longer than 3-5 seconds);

8. Your eyes will be observed again for nystagmus—we call this secondary stage nystagmus (for a successful treatment, this secondary stage nystagmus should beat in the same direction as the primary stage nystagmus);

9. You'll maintain this position for 30-60 seconds and then sit back up (position A)—with a successful maneuver there should be no nystagmus or vertigo when you return to the sitting position.

Some people, such as the elderly, have difficulty moving through the various positions, but especially those with neck and back problems. Such people may not be able to keep their

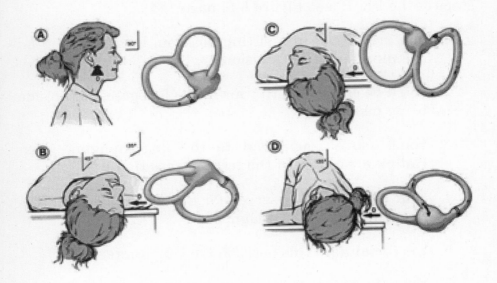

Figure 6-3. Particle Repositioning Maneuver (right ear). Schema of patient and concurrent movement of posterior/superior semicircular canals and utricle. (Explanation on opposite page)

Explaination of Figure 6-3

You would be seated on a table as viewed from the right side (A). The remaining parts show the sequential head and body positions if you were lying down as viewed from the top. Before moving you into position B, you'll be asked to turn your head 45° to the side being treated (in this case it would be the right side). In position B, you'll be in the normal Dix–Hallpike head-hanging position. Particles gravitate in an ampullofugal direction and induce utriculofugal cupular displacement and subsequent counter-clockwise rotatory nystagmus. This position is maintained for 1–2 minutes. Your head is then rotated toward the opposite side with the neck in full extension through position C and into position D in a steady motion by being rolled onto your opposite lateral side. The change from position B to D should take no longer than 3–5 seconds.

Particles continue gravitating in an ampullofugal direction through the common crus into the utricle. Your eyes are immediately observed for nystagmus. If the particles continue moving in the same ampullofugal direction (that is, through the common crus into the utricle), this secondary stage nystagmus should beat in the same direction as the primary stage nystagmus.

Position D is maintained for another 1–2 minutes and then you'll sit back up to position A. With a successful maneuver there should be no nystagmus or vertigo when you return to the sitting position because the particles will have already been repositioned into the utricle.

Position D is the direction of view of the labyrinth; the dark circle is the position of particle conglomerate; and the open circle is the previous position.

necks in full extension as described in step 6 above. Since the purpose of this whole maneuver is to orient and turn the posterior canal in the plane of gravity, one way to get around this is to have a table that tilts backwards, which will eliminate the need for neck extension. Some clinics have special "gyroscope" chairs in which patients are firmly strapped so that they can be turned in any plane in space, even upside down. This more sophisticated type of equipment is not necessary for routine use, and serves more of a research purpose.

Some patients may become nauseated, and even vomit at any time during the procedure. If this happens, the procedure should be aborted and measures should be taken to prevent it from recurring. One such measure is to pre-medicate with an anti-nausea drug prior to the next attempt which might be at the same clinic visit, or at a subsequent visit depending on how ill you feel.

Overall, the PRM should take less than five minutes to complete. Some clinicians will then immediately repeat the Dix-Hallpike maneuver to check for the BPPV response. Others, like me, do only one PRM per visit unless there's reason to believe that it did not work, for example if there are atypical nystagmus responses observed during steps 8 and 9 above. My reason for not immediately repeating the Dix-Hallpike maneuver is to avoid "undoing" a successful PRM, which can happen if the particles re-enter the posterior canal in the "head hanging" position. It's also possible to convert posterior canal BPPV into lateral canal BPPV with repeat testing.

If more than one canal is affected such as both posteriors, or one posterior and one lateral, only one canal should be treated at a time, usually the one causing the most problems. Following the PRM, patients are then typically asked to remain as upright as possible for the following 24-48 hours. Some clinicians simply tell patients not to lay down flat while others insist that patients go so far as to sleep in a chair for the upcoming night or two. Some recommend that patients wear a soft neck collar so that they don't tip their head back. Based on some earlier recommendations, some clinicians still tell patients not to lie on the affected side for up to one week afterwards.

Until recently, my only restriction after the treatment was to recommend not to lie down for 24 hours, but lately, based on recent studies in the medical literature, I have given no post-treatment restrictions. I typically have my patients return to see me approximately three to four weeks after the treatment. At the follow-up visit, I check the treated canal first, and if there is a normal response, I then check the other canals with the Dix-Hallpike test. If need be, a repositioning maneuver is performed on the appropriate canal.

In my experience of performing over 1200 particle repositioning maneuvers, about 80 percent of patients are made significantly better with just one treatment session while about 95 percent can be helped with as many as three treatment sessions. In this latter group of patients that have presumably been "cured" of their BPPV, a significant number will still complain of more vague sensations of imbalance and lightheadedness, even though their Dix-Hallpike test for BPPV is negative. I suspect that these latter patients still experience residual "inner ear" symptoms from the problem that caused the BPPV in the first place, such as the viral inner ear infection, Ménière's disease or inner ear concussion from head trauma. These are the patients who might also benefit from vestibular physiotherapy, as discussed in Chapter 10.

Lateral Canal BPPV

Several positioning techniques have also been developed to treat lateral canal BPPV. Perhaps the most simple is the "prolonged position maneuver" developed by Vannucchi. In lateral BPPV cases that have geotropic nystagmus, the patient lies on their side with the affected ear up for 12 hours. The barrel roll, as described by Dr. Epley, was developed to treat canalithiasis of the lateral semicircular canal. It involves rolling the patient 360º, from flat on the back all away around until they are flat on their back again. What this does is spin the lateral canal around so that the debris gets dumped out of the canal back into the utricle, which is the same concept in treating the more common posterior canal BPPV with the PRM. The patient is rolled away from the affected ear in 90º increments until a full roll is completed and with each change in position, the eyes are observed for the appropriate nystagmus.

Predicting Success and Recurrence Risk

Several studies have attempted to identify variables that would help predict initial short-term success and recurrence risk with repositioning maneuvers. The success of the PRM is not affected by the following factors: the age or sex of the patient; the cause of the BPPV be it primary or secondary; the duration of symptoms before treatment; the presence of recurrent or permanent BPPV before repositioning; the number of repositioning maneuvers performed per treatment visit. However, patients with BPPV affecting both ears or with BPPV in a canal other than the posterior canal do require a greater number of treatment sessions until resolution of symptoms.

BPPV often recurs after successful repositioning. About one third of patients have a recurrence in the first year after treatment, and by five years, as many as half will have a recurrence. In such cases, the BPPV might recur in the original ear or might also occur in the other ear. Regardless, it usually responds readily to another repositioning maneuver. Only rarely does a patient not respond to treatment, or have so many frequent, troublesome recurrences that aggressive surgical treatment would be recommended.

Surgical Treatment

There are various theoretical reasons why repositioning maneuvers might not work. The most important consideration is for the clinician to ensure that the correct diagnosis on the correct canal had been made. If so, surgery should then be considered, but only for the most severely symptomatic cases that don't respond to several repositioning maneuvers, or those that frequently recur. Furthermore, before considering surgery, the inner ear connections with the base of the brain should be assessed with a CT scan or MRI to look for other diseases such as tumors that might mimic BPPV.

Singular Neurectomy

Posterior ampullary nerve section (*singular neurectomy*) was developed by Dr. Richard Gacek in Syracuse, N.Y. in the 1970's. This is the nerve that sends impulses exclusively from the posterior semicircular canal to the balance part of the brain. Although the procedure is highly effective, early reports showed a high rate of hearing loss from damage to the organ of hearing. The procedure is technically demanding even for the most experienced ear surgeon and has largely been replaced by the simpler posterior semicircular canal occlusion.

Posterior Semicircular Canal Occlusion

Dr. Joseph McClure and I were the first to introduce the concept of *posterior semicircular canal occlusion* for BPPV in the 1980s. We proposed, and still feel this to be true, that occluding (plugging) the semicircular canal lumen prevents endolymph flow. This effectively fixes the cupula and makes it unresponsive to both the normal angular acceleration forces and more importantly, the abnormal stimulation from either free-floating particles within the endolymph (canalithiasis) or a fixed cupular deposit (cupulolithiasis). Until the advent of this procedure, invasive inner ear surgery was felt to be too risky in normal hearing ears. However, before performing this procedure in patients with BPPV, we laid the groundwork in an animal experiment by demonstrating its negligible effect on hearing.

In most specialized dizziness clinics around the world, posterior semicircular canal occlusion has become the surgical procedure of choice for unremitting or recurring BPPV. I would not recommend the procedure in an only hearing ear, but otherwise, as long as the patient can tolerate a general anaesthetic, there should be no contraindications (reasons not) to do the surgery. The procedure is done in the hospital operating room under general anaesthetic and should take about two to three hours. The posterior canal is accessed through the mastoid bone. To get to it, the surgeon makes a curved two inch incision through the skin just behind the attachment of the ear. Once it heals up, the scar is mostly hidden by hair and barely noticeable. After exposing the bone under the incision, the mastoid bone is literally drilled away until the structures of the inner ear are identified. Then with the use of an operating microscope, the posterior canal is gently opened up with extreme care taken not to damage the other delicate inner ear structures. The opening into the canal measures about 1 mm across and 3 mm long.

Although other materials may be used, I use a plug, made from some of the bone chips that were drilled away mixed with special tissue glue, to occlude the canal. The drilled out mastoid bone does not have to be replaced since it heals in with scar tissue. The operation is complete once the incision is sutured closed. A tight head wrap dressing is applied and left on for a day or two. Most patients stay in the hospital for two to three days after surgery, the length of which depends on the degree of imbalance they have after surgery. Since, as stated before, the operation affects the normal inner ear function, all patients will have imbalance and sensitivity to movement for some time after surgery. For most people, the brain adapts to this after a few days to a few weeks, with vestibular physiotherapy hastening this process.

The major risks are twofold. First is the risk to hearing. In my own experience in performing this operation in over 40 normal hearing ears, only one patient developed a significant hearing loss following surgery, and this didn't occur until three months later. Unlike all of my other patients, this patient had also undergone two previous unsuccessful singular neurectomies by another surgeon, and this may have complicated matters. The other risk is that of imbalance and motion sensitivity that may go on for months, or even years despite physiotherapy. This happens in about 10 percent of individuals, and is thought to be due to some maladaptive brain condition which unfortunately cannot be identified by any specific tests. Those of my patients that have had this problem still felt better off with this persistent imbalance compared to their pre-surgical positional vertigo. The other potential complications are those that might occur with any operation including infection, bleeding and complications from the anaesthetic.

Summary

Benign paroxysmal positional vertigo presents with a history of brief, episodic, position-provoked vertigo with characteristic findings on Dix-Hallpike testing. Whereas a variety of positional maneuvers have been described, the particle repositioning maneuver is a simple effective treatment for most patients with objective or subjective BPPV. Current evidence does not support the routine use of skull vibration with repositioning. Although most clinicians are still advising patients to remain upright for 24-48 hours after repositioning, recent evidence suggests that this is unnecessary. The recommendation regarding the ideal number of repositioning maneuvers to perform per treatment session varies from clinic to clinic. To date, no factors have been identified to indicate an increased risk of BPPV recurrence after successful repositioning; however, there seems to be some association between BPPV recurrence and migraine. There is an overall long term recurrence risk that may be as high as 50 percent. Fortunately, most of these cases can be successfully treated again with repeat repositioning. For the small group of patients with classic posterior canal BPPV who do not respond to repositioning, posterior canal occlusion is a safe and highly effective procedure.

CHAPTER SEVEN

Ménière's Disease – A Patient's Odyssey

John L. Dornhoffer, MD

Professor and Director of the Division of Otology/Neurotology
University of Arkansas for Medical Sciences
Executive Director of the Prosper Ménière Society

Dr. Dornhoffer is Professor and Director of the Division of Otology/Neurotology at the University of Arkansas for Medical Sciences and Executive Director of the Prosper Ménière Society. Dr. Dornhoffer's goal is to restore hearing in as many individuals as possible, and a major research interest centers around Ménière's Disease. Dr. Dornhoffer sees approximately 500 patients with this condition each year, and his research centers around understanding fluid control in the inner ear in Ménière's disease. Dr. Dornhoffer has over 60 publications, several patents relating to ear surgery, and is a member of the Triological Society, the American Otologic Society, and the American Neurotology Society.

Ménière's disease gets its name from Prosper Ménière, a French physician who in 1861 first attributed a condition linking tinnitus and vertigo to a disorder of the inner ear. Today, Ménière's disease is described as a syndrome comprising four classic symptoms: hearing loss, vertigo (dizziness), tinnitus (a roaring or ringing sound in the ear) and aural fullness (a feeling of pressure in the ear, as if the ear is plugged and the eardrum needs to be "popped"). Two variants of classical Ménière's disease include only three of the four symptoms. Patients with Cochlear Ménière's disease do not experience the vertigo but do have the other symptoms of hearing loss, tinnitus and aural fullness. Patients with Vestibular Ménière's disease experience the vertigo, tinnitus and aural fullness but do not have any hearing loss. Because it's a collection of symptoms, Ménière's disease is often called Ménière's syndrome, which may actually be the more accurate term.

Susan, a wife and mother of two, was 31 years of age when her symptoms first appeared. She woke up from a nap and everything was spinning. This episode of vertigo lasted for over an hour, making her feel weak and sick with nausea. A few days later, the dizziness attacked again although it subsided more quickly and didn't seem as severe. Susan then started to notice a roaring sound in her right ear, as if a waterfall was cascading through her head. She also had a feeling of pressure in the same ear, the same feeling she had when she was flying and the airplane started to descend. Not linking these symptoms with her dizzy attacks, Susan thought she had an ear infection since she had been plagued by these as a young child. However, she had no feelings of pain in her ear and a short round of antibiotics seemed to make no difference.

Ménière's Symptoms

The symptoms of Ménière's disease typically appear in individuals between the ages of 30 and 50 years, but there are many exceptions to this. Ménière's disease is actually a rare condition. According to the National Institutes of Health List of Rare Diseases, there are less than 200,000 cases in the U.S. Some researchers have described Ménière's disease as being familial, meaning it can run in families, particularly when the symptoms are associated with migraine headaches. It is estimated that 10-15 percent of patients experience bilateral Ménière's disease, with symptoms occurring in both ears.

Susan made an appointment with her family physician. Although her attacks of vertigo were never quite as severe as the first one she had experienced, they were still occurring on a fairly frequent basis. She was becoming afraid to drive, especially when her children were in the car, because she might experience a dizzy attack. In addition, the feeling of pressure (or aural fullness) was now occurring more fre-

quently. She had nearly convinced herself of the worst-case scenario—a brain tumor. Fortunately, her family physician was able to calm her fears. He thought she was still experiencing an ear infection and explained that an ear infection could also cause disequilibrium (dizziness). He prescribed cortisone to reduce any swelling in the inner ear and relieve the pressure, as well as a different round of antibiotics to clear up the infection. Susan left the doctor's office confident that all her symptoms would soon be going away.

The symptoms of Ménière's disease can pose as many other illnesses, causing frustration, anxiety and depression in the patient suffering from this disease as he or she tries to cope with the attacks of vertigo while attempting to determine the cause. Until a diagnosis is confirmed, many patients start to feel as if they're going crazy and their family and colleagues may even accuse them of shirking work duties and faking symptoms.

Although Susan's symptoms are frequently diagnosed as an inner ear infection, this is unlikely to be the cause. An inner ear infection is either due to bacteria (bacterial labyrinthitis) or a virus (vestibular neuronitis). However, true bacterial labyrinthitis is extremely rare and would cause complete deafness whereas vestibular neuronitis would typically occur only once, causing a single episode of vertigo and no hearing loss or tinnitus. In addition, because vestibular neuronitis is caused by a virus, antibiotics would be of no help. Unfortunately, an inner ear infection is a common misdiagnosis for patients facing the first signs of Ménière's disease.

There are many other diseases or conditions with symptoms similar to Ménière's disease, including acoustic neuroma, multiple sclerosis, aneurysms, cerebellar or brainstem tumors, benign paroxysmal positional vertigo, perilymphatic fistula, otosclerosis, diabetes, syphilis, anemia and autoimmune disorders.

In Susan's case, her relief was short-lived. Not long after completing the second series of antibiotics, she was visiting with a friend when a dizzy attack literally dropped her to the floor. The room was spinning so badly she began to vomit from the nausea. Thinking she was having a seizure, Susan's friend drove her to the emergency room where she was monitored closely for any other attacks. An EEG (electroencephalogram) showed that nothing was wrong with her brain activity and she was sent home with a prescription for meclizine (a drug used to treat vertigo). Exhausted by her ordeal, Susan went to bed although it was only mid-afternoon and slept until the next morning.

Vertigo, the feeling that the room is spinning, is surely the most debilitating symptom of Ménière's disease. The degree of vertigo experienced by individuals varies considerably. Some may experience mild dizziness while others experience acute attacks of severe dizziness that last anywhere from a few minutes to a few hours. Some individuals are able to predict an oncoming attack of vertigo. The "drop attack" experienced by Susan represents the most severe type of vertigo described by patients with Ménière's disease. In such cases, the individual literally drops to the ground—thus the name—because the sudden onset of vertigo is so overwhelming. The individual feels helpless as the world literally spins out of control. The sudden motion often causes severe nausea to the point of vomiting. After the attack subsides, the individual may sleep for hours or days.

Several weeks passed and Susan experienced no more vertigo. In fact, the feeling of aural fullness also seemed to go away. However, after a month of being symptom-free, Susan began again to experience pressure and tinnitus in her right ear. A repeat drop attack sent her back to her family physician for a complete work-up.

The symptoms of Ménière's disease fluctuate. In other words, the intensity and duration of the vertigo, tinnitus, aural fullness and hearing loss will vary within an individual, with no consistent pattern linking their severity or extent. The symptoms may not even occur at the same time; some will be severe while others are mild; or there may be periods during the course of the disease when there are no symptoms at all. Thus, Ménière's disease is often described as "episodic," with patients experiencing periods of complete relief from all symptoms, particularly during early stages of the disease.

In addition, the symptoms manifest differently in different patients. Some patients experience frequent acute drop attacks while others describe only mild feelings of dizziness. The descriptions of tinnitus run the gamut from a constant chirping noise or roaring sound to intermittent episodes of thumping or a loud whine. Some patients experience the feeling of aural fullness to the point of pain whereas, in others, this symptom remains relatively mild. Finally, some patients with Ménière's disease quickly lose their hearing in the affected ear while others lose their hearing more slowly and never to the point of complete deafness. However, the extent of hearing loss increases over time in the majority of patients. This variability in the occurrence and severity of the four symptoms adds to the confusion when trying to diagnosis and treat patients with Ménière's disease.

Testing for Ménière's Disease

Ménière's disease remains the purview of the otolaryngologist. In particular, a *neurotologist* (subspecialty ear surgeon) or *otoneurologist* (a medical neurologist specializing in balance disorders) will diagnose and manage patients with Ménière's disease. In fact, many of the additional tests used to diagnose a patient with Ménière's disease are only performed at centers that specifically treat patients with balance disorders.

Susan soon began the odyssey of testing and refer-rals. An EKG (electrocardiogram) and Tilt Table test showed nothing was wrong with her heart. A CT (computerized tomography) scan and visit to a neurologist indicated that she had not experienced a stroke and did not have a tumor or anything else wrong with her brain. Her electrolytes and CBC (complete blood count) came back normal. Lacking any other findings, Susan's physician referred her to an otolaryngologist.

Dr. Davis, Susan's neurotologist, ordered additional blood tests, an MRI and a series of audiologic tests. These included an audiogram and ENG. He also performed a balance assessment using a rotary chair and performed posturography and electrocochleography.

The diagnosis of Ménière's disease is a diagnosis of exclusion. In other words, the neurotologist must first rule out, or exclude, other possible causes of the symptoms before the diagnosis of Ménière's disease can be made. Thus, the neurotologist will order both serologic (blood) and audiologic (ear) tests. Typical blood tests include an erythrocyte (red blood cell) sedimentation rate, an ANA (antinuclear antibody) test and rheumatoid factor to determine if an autoimmune disease is the cause of the patient's symptoms, and thyroid function tests to determine if hypo- or hyperthyroidism is a cause of the vertigo. Tests may also be ordered to assess cholesterol levels since high cholesterol can impair hearing and mimic Ménière's disease. A VDRL (Venereal Disease Research Laboratory) test and an FTA/ABS (fluorescent treponemal antibody absorption) test are traditionally ordered to rule out syphilis, known as the "old masquerader" of Ménière's disease. Patients with Ménière's-like symptoms are routinely screened for syphilis and should not feel insulted when this test is ordered.

If a patient has not already had one, an MRI with a contrast agent such as gadolinium will be ordered to rule out an acoustic neuroma since this can be missed with a CT scan. Acoustic neuromas are slow-growing, usually benign tumors that can grow on the vestibular nerve and cause Ménière's-like symptoms.

Typical audiologic tests include an audiogram and ENG. An audiogram (basic hearing test) will determine if the patient has any hearing loss and, if so, at what frequencies. With ENG (electronystagmography or caloric stimulation test), warm water and then cold water is placed in the patient's outer ear canal to induce vertigo. The patient's eyes are then observed and a weakness in the affected ear is indicated if nystagmus (a rapid side-to-side eye movement) is seen.

Additional tests can also be performed, particularly when the diagnosis is difficult. Some of these have previously been discussed in Chapter 3. The *rotational chair test* assesses inner ear function. Another test is posturography in which the patient's balance reaction is observed when standing on a platform that moves. This is a functional assessment of how a patient's eyes, ears, and joints interact to maintain balance. A PLF test (perilymphatic fistula) can determine if there's a hole in the membrane between the middle ear and inner ear by applying positive and negative pressure to the ear canal. A perilymphatic fistula is indicated if the test causes nystagmus and vertigo.

Electrocochleography may also be ordered to indirectly measure fluid pressure in the inner ear. With electrocochleography (ECoG) a sensor is placed in the outer ear canal and the electrical response of the inner ear to clicking sounds is recorded. There are a number of abnormal ECoG results associated with Ménière's disease and if these are present on the ECoG tracing, Ménière's disease is indicated. However, if electrocochleography is negative, the results are not definitive and one cannot rule out a diagnosis of Ménière's disease. For this reason, electrocochleography is not always ordered with the first battery of tests.

Although not performed as frequently as in the past primarily due to a number of unpleasant side effects, the *glycerol dehydration test* may be given to obtain a diagnosis. In this test, the patient ingests glycerol mixed with an equal amount of water or juice in an effort to dehydrate the system (and thus relieve the inner ear fluid pressure caused by the Ménière's disease). A hearing test is then administered three hours later. If the hearing test shows an improvement in hearing, the patient is likely to have Ménière's disease.

When Susan met with Dr. Davis at the conclusion of her tests, she was very nervous. What if everything was normal—again! Was she imagining her symptoms? Was she becoming a hypochondriac? Susan was afraid Dr. Davis would have nothing more to tell her and that she would have to continue with more tests and more frustration. So it was with relief that she heard his diagnosis.

"Susan," Dr. Davis told her, "based on your history of symptoms and the fact that the majority of your tests came back normal, I'm confident you have a disease called Ménière's disease. Your MRI showed no acoustic neuroma and your blood tests indicate no thyroid disease or autoimmune disorders. Your audiogram, which was the only test with an abnormal finding, indicated a sensorineural hearing loss in the low tones. This means you have had damage to your hearing nerve and will likely have a harder time understanding what is being spoken to you."

"But how can we be sure if all the other tests are negative?" Susan asked.

Dr. Davis smiled. "That's a very good question. Like yourself, many patients with Ménière's disease will have no symptoms at the time their diagnostic tests are administered and, therefore, their test results will all come back normal. Half the patients with Ménière's disease will have a normal ENG. In fact, the hearing test may also come back normal in between episodes of the disease and before it has progressed. You have Stage Two Ménière's disease because you exhibit a hearing loss even though you are not currently suffering a Ménière's attack."

Because many of the audiologic tests will come back negative, the neurotologist will often make the diagnosis of
Ménière's disease based on the patient's history and symptom
complex and after ruling out all other possibilities (the diagnosis of exclusion). The typical symptom complex the neurotologist will rely on to make the final diagnosis is a low-tone
sensorineural hearing loss, tinnitus that is typically in the low
tones and "roaring," and episodes of vertigo that last 10 minutes to 24 hours.

The Stages of Ménière's Disease

Ménière's disease is classified into four stages. A patient
with Stage One disease experiences episodic vertigo with
episodic hearing loss that returns to normal between attacks.
A patient with Stage Two disease has episodic vertigo with
hearing loss that improves but does not return to normal
between attacks. In Stage Three disease, the patient has
episodic vertigo and a "flat" sensorineural hearing loss—a loss
at both the low and high frequencies. In Stage Four Ménière's
disease, the hearing no longer fluctuates and the vertigo has
gone away leaving the patient with some disequilibrium. This
is known as "burned-out" Ménière's disease.

"What causes Ménière's disease?" Susan asked.

*Dr. Davis explained. "The inner ear is much like a
sink filled with fluid. The fluid in the inner ear is
called endolymph and it's produced by a structure in
the cochlea called the stria vascularis. The endolymph
flows through the cochlea to the endolymphatic sac
which drains the fluid."* (See Figure 7-1)

*"So, this stria vascularis is the faucet, the cochlea
is the sink and the endolymphatic sac is the drain?"
asked Susan.*

*"Correct!" said Dr. Davis. "And with Ménière's dis-
ease there's a problem with the drain. Since the
drain—the endolylmphatic sac— is plugged up or not
working, the fluid builds up in the cochlea. This causes the symptoms of Ménière's disease."*

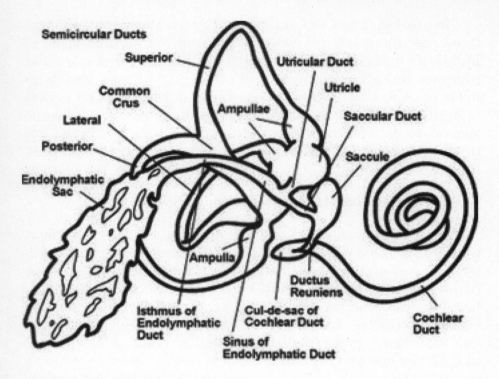

Figure 7-1: Endolymphatic System

The ear can be divided into three sections: the external ear which is the visible portion of the ear including the ear canal and ending with the tympanic membrane (eardrum); the middle ear where the three ear bones (the hammer or malleus, the anvil or incus, and the stirrup or stapes) reside; and the inner ear or labyrinth. The labyrinth contains the structures that help control hearing and balance. These include the cochlea, the three semicircular canals and the vestibule which contains the Otolith organs (the utricle and saccule). The endolymphatic sac lies outside the labyrinth and contains endolymph—a sodium-rich fluid found only in the inner ear.

The endolymphatic sac is involved in fluid regulation in the inner ear and it can both produce and absorb endolymph. It is currently believed that dysfunction of the endolymphatic sac leads to a build-up of endolymph called *endolymphatic hydrops* (elevated endolymph fluid pressure) which in turn causes symptoms of Ménière's disease. Some researchers believe the drop attacks experienced by patients with Ménière's disease are caused by the sudden flow of fluid into the endolymphatic sac, producing a rupture of Reissner's membrane in the cochlea and causing endolymph to leak into perilymph, a potassium-rich inner ear fluid, or into the labyrinth, where it interferes with the tiny hairs that are involved with hearing and balance. However, the cause of the dysfunction of the endolymphatic sac or of the build-up of fluid is not known. Thus, Ménière's disease and the associated endolymphatic hydrops are described as idiopathic (of unknown cause).

Medical Treatment

To control her symptoms, Susan's doctor prescribed a low sodium diet and Maxzide,™ a diuretic. He also instructed her to keep a diary of her symptoms, particularly any attacks of vertigo. She was instructed to avoid caffeine, alcohol, tobacco and stress since these could bring on an attack. She was to make a follow-up appointment in three months.

Until the cause of Ménière's disease can be determined there can be no actual cure. Instead, the patient with Ménière's disease is treated for the symptoms, particularly for the vertigo, rather than for the underlying disease. In the U.S., first-line treatment to prevent vertigo consists of a low sodium diet of 2000 mg sodium per day plus a diuretic, such as Maxzide™ or Dyazide™ (triamterene with hydrochlorothiazide), Lasix™ (furosemide) or Bumex™ (bumetanide). A low sodium diet means the patient must avoid salty foods, must not add table salt when preparing foods, must not add salt to prepared foods, and must count milligrams of sodium that can occur naturally in foods or be added as a preservative (see the Low Sodium table in Chapter Eight, page 179). Salt substitutes are discouraged unless discussed with your doctor. Pepper and other spices are excellent alternatives. It is believed this combination of a low sodium diet and a diuretic, which will help reduce bodily fluids, will also reduce the excess endolymph. In Europe and Canada, first-line treatment often comprises histamine analogs such as Serc™ (betahistine). Front-line treatment is initiated even if a patient's tests are normal but he or she has a history of the symptoms of Ménière's disease.

The Ménière's patient will also be instructed to keep a diary of any vertigo episodes including details on how long they last, how severe they are and what the patient was doing when an attack occurred. In this way, and in conjunction with follow-up hearing tests, the physician and patient can track improvement or worsening of the disease.

Finally, patients are instructed to avoid CATS. This is not the furry house pet. Rather, the acronym stands for the specific triggers that can bring on an attack of the disease: caffeine, alcohol, tobacco and stress. Other stressors that can bring on the symptoms and should be avoided if possible include both food and seasonal allergies; changes in barometric pressure; and certain visual stimuli, particularly those with parallel vertical lines such as streets lined with trees or telephone poles, supermarket aisles and certain movies.

At her three-month follow-up appointment, Susan was to the point of tears. "I was doing so well," she told Dr. Davis. "I followed the low sodium diet to the letter. My symptoms had virtually disappeared. Then, two weeks ago I had another dizzy spell. It lasted several hours and I was so weak the next day I couldn't go to work. I just started a new job and I'm afraid I'll get fired if I miss much more work!"

"For starters," said Dr. Davis, "I think that new job may have been the problem." He explained, "Major life changes can be extremely stressful. This added stress in your life may have precipitated your attack. You simply let the CAT out of the bag, so to speak. However, all is not lost. After we reassess your hearing, I'm going to give you a prescription for Ativan.™ Now, this is only to be used during an attack to help

treat the vertigo. We'll maintain the salt-free diet and diuretic to control the symptoms and hopefully as you adjust to your new job, this added stress will go away."

Although the patient with Ménière's disease may eventually learn how to cope and "work through" minor spells of vertigo, major attacks such as drop attacks are totally disabling. For this reason, vestibular suppressants, such as Antivert™ or Bonine™ (meclizine hydrochloride), Ativan™ (lorazepam), and Valium™ (diazepam), are often prescribed because once an attack begins, it cannot be stopped and must run its course. These treatments help by suppressing (sedating or blocking) the vestibular apparatus in the inner ear, thus preventing it from sending signals of dizziness to the brain. They also help by controlling the nausea and vomiting that accompany a vertigo attack although they may also have a sedating effect. A mistake is made when a patient begins to take vestibular suppressants constantly since these are intended as "rescue" therapy only, with the diet and diuretic used to control the disease on a chronic basis. This confusion over their use often leads to further problems in the patient with Ménière's disease as these drugs can be habit-forming and can cause drowsiness.

Dr. Davis looked over Susan's diary and follow-up audiogram. It was now six months since her initial diagnosis. Unfortunately, although she diligently avoided the specific triggers, her diary indicated that her vertigo episodes had increased in frequency. Her hearing loss had progressed slightly as well. She now had a 40-dB loss which represented a low-tone hearing loss;,and a 60 percent speech discrimination score. Because Susan's hearing was still in a useful range, Dr. Davis recommended a procedure called endolymphatic shunt surgery (to be discussed in a moment)— an operation to control her attacks of vertigo.

Approximately 80-90 percent of patients with Ménière's disease do well with first-line treatment, experiencing relief of all symptoms for months or even years. Although the low sodium diet/diuretic combination can be continued indefinitely, some patients will forego this treatment if they are symptom-free for one year. Unfortunately, a certain percent of patients experience no relief of symptoms with first-line treatment. In these patients, stepwise treatments are available to relieve the symptoms of vertigo, and these are dictated by the patient's level of hearing. These therapies, many of which are surgical, are typically performed by a neurotologist. Some require hospitalization, but others can be performed in an outpatient setting.

Procedures for Ménière's Disease

If a patient's hearing is normal or good enough to be preserved (<50 dB pure-tone-average loss; >50 percent speech discrimination score), the following treatments are considered.

1. **Endolymphatic sac decompression with or without shunt placement.** Surgical decompression of the sac is considered by many to be the treatment of choice for patients who experience no relief of their symptoms with the low sodium/diuretic regimen. While the patient is under general anesthesia the ear surgeon makes an incision behind the ear to expose the mastoid (the bony sinus behind the ear) and reveal the endolymphatic sac. The bone covering the endolymphatic sac is removed to decompress the sac. In addition, a shunt (tiny tube) may be positioned into the sac. The theory is that the shunt will be able to drain off the excess endolymph. About half of the decompression surgeries utilize the shunt and results seem to be the same whether or not a shunt is used. The advantages of this treatment are that it's simple (the patient can undergo the surgery as an outpatient) and it preserves the hearing. The disadvantage is the success rate. Although 75 percent of patients report significant control of vertigo

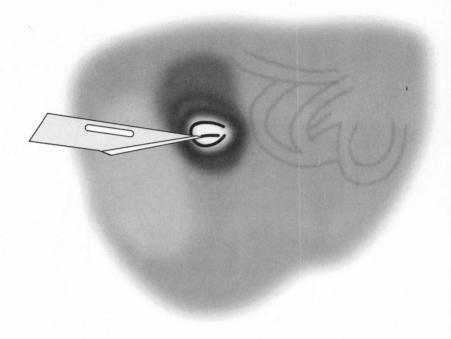

Figure 7-2: Endolymphatic Sac Decompression

at one year after the surgery, at five years, only 50 percent of patients experience continued relief (see Figure
7-2).

2. **Vestibular nerve section (VNS) or vestibular neurectomy.** With this surgical procedure, which is performed
under general anesthetic, the neurotologist makes an
incision behind the ear and enters the skull between
the brain and the ear in order to severe the vestibular
(balance) nerve. Thus, the nerve will no longer be able
to send "dizzy" signals to the brain. The advantage of
this procedure is that it's 90 percent effective in controlling vertigo. However, it has several disadvantages. It
can cause some mild permanent imbalance in the
patient; it's invasive; and, because it's an intracranial

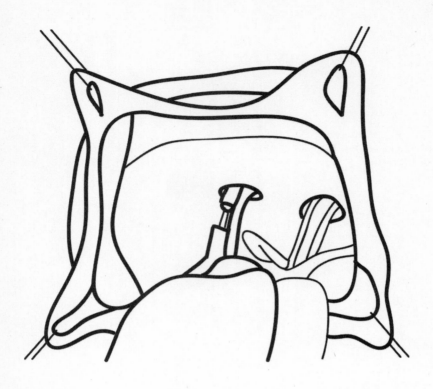

Figure 7-3: Vestibular Nerve Section (VNS)

procedure (brain surgery), the patient will require hospitalization including one night in the intensive care unit. There's also a slight risk of facial nerve injury and hearing loss with this procedure (see Figure 7-3).

3. **Meniett™ Low-Pressure Pulse Generator (Medtronic Xomed, Inc.).** The Meniett represents a relatively new method for alleviating the symptoms of Ménière's disease. This portable device consists of a small tube that has a nipple at one end and is attached to a pulse generator at the other end (see Figure 7-4). After having a tube inserted through the eardrum (much like the pressure equalizing tubes used in children to control ear

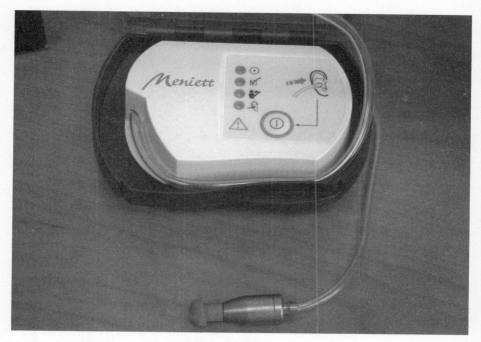

Figure 7-4: Meniett™ Low-Pressure Pulse Generator

infections), the patient uses the Meniett to apply positive pressure to the ear for five minutes, three times a
day. This positive pressure causes displacement of
inner ear fluids. It's believed that this restores the
inner ear fluid dynamics, thereby relieving the
endolymphatic hydrops and symptoms of Ménière's disease. This is an easy treatment that can be performed
at home. Although results are encouraging (a multicen-
ter study in Europe has shown that good control of vertigo can be obtained with the device), results in the U.S.
are still preliminary. (More information is available on
page 225.)

4. **Dexamethasone perfusion.** This treatment involves
applying topical anesthetic to the eardrum, making a
hole in the eardrum with a needle or laser, and instill-
ing the steroid dexamethasone into the middle ear
space in an effort to reduce inflammation and suppress
the immune system. A microwick, microcatheter or

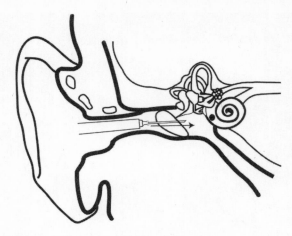

Figure 7-5: Dexamethasone Perfusion

piece of absorbable gelatin can also be used to deliver the treatment to the round window. The perfusion is usually repeated with a series of multiple injections performed several days in a row. Dexamethasone perfusion is considered experimental and results are controversial. Although good results have been reported by some, others claim to have a poor control of vertigo with this treatment (see Figure 7-5).

5. **Intramuscular streptomycin.** Since streptomycin affects the vestibular system without affecting hearing, it can be given to those patients who have bilateral Ménière's disease, where both ears are affected, or to patients who have Ménière's disease in an only-hearing ear. The drug is given by injection into the muscle twice a day for five days, after which time the patient's symptoms and hearing level are re-evaluated. If symptoms persist, injections are given for another three days. Two-day treatments are continued every two weeks until symptoms disappear or if hearing worsens.

Susan recovered well from her endolymphatic shunt surgery. However, by three months, her vertigo episodes returned. She had a hearing loss of 50 dB in her right ear and a 50 percent speech discrimination

*score. Because Susan's hearing had worsened, Dr.
Davis recommended gentamicin perfusion over the
next three weeks.*

*"We'll know in a few weeks if the therapy worked,"
he told her. "However, there's a risk that your hearing
may actually get worse."*

*"I don't even care about my hearing any more,"
she told Dr. Davis. "I just want to get rid of these vertigo spells. I can't work. I can't take care of my two little boys. I can't do anything if I'm dizzy all the time!"*

In many patients with Ménière's disease, the hearing has
deteriorated to such an extent that hearing preservation is no
longer a consideration. In others, as in Susan's case, hearing
preservation therapies don't work to control the vertigo. For
all these patients, other treatment options are available.

1. **Surgical labyrinthectomy**. With this procedure, which
is performed under general anesthesia, the neurotologist
makes an incision through the mastoid and drills away the
labyrinth, which contains the balance organs of the inner ear,
until it is destroyed. The brain no longer receives dizzy signals
from the affected ear and the unaffected ear takes over the
balance function for both ears. This is a simple and straight-
forward procedure and effectively controls vertigo in 90 percent of the patients who undergo it, although some mild disequilibrium may be experienced. The disadvantage of this procedure is that it destroys any possibility of preserving hearing
in the treated ear. Although this doesn't matter if the hearing
has already deteriorated in that ear, it will limit the treatment options if the disease progresses to the other ear. There
is also a slight risk of facial nerve injury with this procedure.

2. **Gentamicin perfusion** (chemical labyrinthectomy).
Gentamicin is one of the aminoglycosides, which are
toxic to the inner ear. After applying topical anesthetic,
the neurotologist uses a needle to inject the gentamicin
through the eardrum into the middle ear space where
it's absorbed through the round window into the inner

ear. A laser may also be used to form the hole in the eardrum through which a piece of absorbable gelatin soaked in the drug can be placed at the round window. A microwick or microcatheter may also be used to deliver the drug. After several treatments, usually three spaced one week apart, the vestibule (the inner ear organ that controls balance) is slowly damaged and the vertigo goes away. The other ear then compensates for the loss of balance, as with a surgical labyrinthectomy described above. The advantages of gentamicin perfusion are that it does not require surgery (and can be performed in a doctor's office, exam room or outpatient setting) and it is able to control vertigo in 90 percent of patients. In addition, there's no risk to the facial nerve. The disadvantages are that it causes an increased incidence of further hearing loss in 5-30 percent of patients. Thus, it is usually considered in patients who have already experienced a substantial loss of hearing.

Compensating for Your Loss of Inner Ear Function

The gentamicin perfusion therapy appeared to work for Susan. Unfortunately, as a side effect of the therapy, she experienced a feeling of being off-balance or unsteady. She had to teach her body how to cope with just one balance system—the one in her left ear. Therefore, soon after her gentamicin therapy was completed, her doctor referred her to a vestibular rehab team. They gave her specific exercises to perform to improve her balance, including several exercises to improve her balance-eye coordination (vestibulo-ocular reflex—VOR) and her standing and walking balance.

The imbalance experienced by patients undergoing surgical or chemical labyrinthectomy is due to the intended destruction of the vestibule, which is necessary to get rid of the symptoms of vertigo. It is easier for the body to adapt to a complete vestibular loss in one ear than a fluctuating or partial loss, as is present in Ménière's disease. The body compensates in time, a process helped by vestibular rehabilitation and the performance of specific exercises designed to stimulate and promote adaptation of the VOR and "train" the body to maintain balance with just one vestibular system.

By her three-month follow-up visit, Susan had experienced no more attacks of vertigo and was regaining her sense of balance. A hearing test showed her hearing loss had stabilized at 50 dB. Dr. Davis discussed getting a hearing aid. "You may not want to wear the hearing aid all the time," he told her. "Your hearing is normal in your left ear, but with your poor speech discrimination, wearing a hearing aid in your right ear may just sound like you've turned up a broken speaker."

The problem with having a single hearing ear is that sound amplification in the worse ear may distort perceived hearing. Turning up a broken speaker is a good analogy since the hearing aid may only amplify sounds that are poorly perceived to begin with. However, individuals may still gain benefit from a hearing aid for non-speech sounds. In those 10-15 percent of patients who experience the disease in both ears, a cochlear implant to restore hearing in one of the affected ears is also an option.

Susan did find the hearing aid was hard to adjust to, especially when trying to hear conversations. However, she enjoyed wearing it to hear background sounds, like the first birds of spring and her children's laughter. And thankfully the vertigo attacks appeared to be gone for good. She felt as if her two-year-long odyssey was at last at an end.

Research and Hope for the Future

Unfortunately, even with more advanced treatments, Ménière's disease is progressive, with patients experiencing a worsening of symptoms over time. Much research into this disease has thus focused on the etiology since it's only by determining the cause of Ménière's disease that a true cure will be obtained.

One line of research is exploring inner ear pharmacokinetics in order to determine:

1. What drugs are the most useful as therapy for Ménière's disease?
2. What's the best method for delivering the drug?
3. How much of the drug should be delivered?

Research is also examining the cause of the disease. Several possibilities have been proposed, including:

1. Allergy
2. Autoimmune origins
3. Genetic inheritance
4. Viral infection
5. Head trauma or prolonged exposure to loud noise

Contributor's Note and Summary

Susan and her physician, whose experiences have been highlighted in this chapter, are fictitious. Her ordeal was drawn out in order to illustrate the stepwise approach to treating Ménière's disease. Fortunately, the majority of Ménière's patients are able to control their symptoms without having to resort to the multiple treatments Susan had to undergo. By following the stepwise approach to therapy, it is possible to eventually control the vertigo, although many times at the expense of hearing. Research is the key and it's only through further research into the cause of this disease that we can hope to find a cure.

CHAPTER EIGHT

Medical and Neurological
Management of Dizziness

Michael D. Seidman, M.D., FACS
Department of Otolaryngology – Head and Neck Surgery
Henry Ford Health System
West Bloomfield, MI

Nadir Ahmad, M.D.
Department of Otolaryngology – Head and Neck Surgery
Henry Ford Health System
West Bloomfield, MI

Dr. Seidman is the Director-Division of Otologic/Neurotologic Surgery in the Department of Otolaryngology-Head and Neck Surgery for the Henry Ford Health System [HFHS], Director of Otolaryngology Research Laboratory, Co-Director of the Tinnitus Center, Chair of the Complementary/Integrative Medicine Program for HFHS, CEO of Body Language Vitamin Company, and past President of the Michigan Otolaryngology Society. He is Co-Editor of the International Tinnitus Journal, on the Editorial Review Board of seven major Otolaryngology Journals, and of The Journal for Traditional Chinese Medicine. Dr. Seidman has more than 80 major publications to his credit.

Dr. Ahmad is a 3rd year ENT resident at Henry Ford Hospital and has aspirations of becoming a leading authority in the field of Otology. He hails from a family of otolaryngologists. He hopes to one day return to his native homeland of Pakistan where there is a dearth of well-trained otologists. His major influences are his father, Nasir Ahmad, an otolaryngologist in Flint, MI and his mentor, Michael Seidman. Dr. Ahmad is passionate about soccer, his family and his wife, Sophia. He currently resides in Birmingham, MI.

The treatment of dizziness and balance disturbances is often challenging and can be met with frustration by both the physician and you the patient. An often cited statistic is that out of 100 patients with dizziness, a diagnosis is only made in about half despite a careful evaluation. For the other half, doctors often shrug their shoulders, apologize and tell them that we simply don't know why they have this problem.

You must realize that even after a detailed history, examination and testing, we often cannot tell you what precisely is wrong. But do not dismay or lose hope! Over the past several years, many promising new approaches and therapies to treat dizziness have been discovered and are now used routinely in many places all over the world. Our aim is to inform you not only of the medications that have been traditionally used to treat or help with the symptoms of dizziness and vertigo, but also to highlight and consider some of the new and novel, non-traditional therapies. This discussion of various medical treatments, both conventional and alternative, will help you navigate through the complex maze of therapies that are available.

Dizziness can mean many things to many different people. The patient who suffers from dizziness can be referring to such feelings as lightheadedness, unsteadiness, confusion, giddiness or nausea. Other descriptions include a sensation of being pulled, a sensation of walking on a waterbed, a floating sensation, a feeling of being on a boat or just getting off a roller coaster. Typically, describing the sensation that they are experiencing is very difficult for most people with balance problems. To better understand treatments, let's take a quick review of how treatments are related to causes. Table 8-1 will provide you with a good overview of both causes and treatments.

Now that you're aware of many of the different causes of dizziness and vertigo, let's get down to the real nitty-gritty and find out what's out there to treat this annoying, troubling and often times debilitating problem.

Low Sodium Diet for Ménière's Disease

Restriction of dietary salt is very often advised as a first-line therapy to alleviate symptoms of vertigo in Ménière's disease. Because of its apparent success in many patients, a strict low salt (that is, low sodium) diet with a daily allowance

Table 8-1. Common Causes of Vertigo

Disease	Cause	Symptoms	Patient Profile	Medical Treatment
Ménière's Disease	Endolymphatic hydrops (increased endolymph in inner ear)	Sudden onset of vertigo, tinnitus, fluctuating sensorineural hearing loss, ear fullness	20-60 yrs old. Typically one ear involved but in 20%, both sides affected	Treatment options diverse. Initial: salt-restricted diet, often in combination with diuretic.
Vestibular Neuronitis	Likely viral infection	Sudden onset disabling vertigo with associated nausea & vomiting, without ear symptoms. Worsens with head motion	Affects any age, sometimes preceded by a viral upper respiratory tract infection.	Symptomatic treatment. Vestibular suppressants (meclizine or diazepam) and antiemetics for relief of intense vertigo, nausea and vomiting in the acute phase. Short-term steroid use also effective
Benign Positional Vertigo (BPV)	Disruption of inner ear crystals	Whirling vertigo induced by specific head position or movement	Most common over age of 40. Females more commonly affected	Symptomatic treatment. Vestibular suppressants for acute phase. Head and/or vestibular exercises to reduce symptoms or a particle repositioning maneuver to reduce symptoms
Perilymphatic fistula	Abnormal connection between inner and middle ear spaces	Symptoms similar to Ménière's	Usually occurs after surgery or trauma	Mainstay is bedrest for 7-10 days. Vestibular suppressants for acute phase.

of 1500-2000 mg of sodium per day is advised. Some doctors advise as low as 1000-1500 mg per day. Although this is very stringent and unpalatable for many people, it has helped many sufferers of dizziness. Perhaps a more reasonable approach but not always effective is to ask patients to avoid excessively salty foods (like highly salted popcorn or crackers) and not add table salt to foods when they're being prepared or served. This more practical approach will result in better compliance and more enjoyable eating. Note the sodium levels in food in Table 8-2.

The thought behind dietary restriction is that less overall fluid will be present in the area of the ear responsible for the symptoms of Ménière's disease. This area called the endolymphatic sac gets enlarged, a condition known as *hydrops*, and is because either too much fluid is getting into the sac or not enough fluid is getting out. The result is what you perceive as spinning or turning, or just plain dizziness.

Restriction in the intake of caffeine, chocolate and alcohol is also recommended for patients with Ménière's disease. In addition, there have been reports that yeast-free and sugar-free diets also help alleviate the symptoms of vertigo. Some patients report that by limiting these substances their attacks occur less frequently. But there is no scientific data to support these claims. The most important thing we advise is that with any form of dietary restriction make sure you determine what is appropriate for you.

For example, if dietary restriction is not working to reduce the symptoms of dizziness, then don't adopt an even more restrictive diet. Your cause of dizziness may not necessarily just respond to diet. A better approach is an objective one. Make a diary of your symptoms, rate the severity and its association to what you eat and do during the day. Don't make strong conclusions right away. Monitor your symptoms over a period of time and decide with the help of your ear doctor which dietary restriction actually makes a difference to your symptoms.

Table 8-2: Sodium Table (measured in mgs./100 gms. edible portion)

Table salt	38,758	Corned beef, cooked	1,740
Bouillon cubes	24,000	Pancake mix, dry	1,433
Baking powder		Pretzels	1,688
w/pyrophosphate	16,804	Ham, sliced	1,429
Teriyaki sauce	10,400	Pickles	
Soup, dehydrated dry		dill	1,428
onion	8,957	sour	1,353
chicken noodle	8,391	Bread stuffing	1,331
clam chowder	7,070	Mustard	
veg. beef	6,460	brown	1,307
tomato veg.	6,722	yellow	1,252
cream of veg.	4,957	Biscuit mix, dry	1,300
mushroom	4,681	Oats, puffed	
minestrone	4,620	nutrients added	1,267
tomato	3,319	Soda crackers	1,100
pea	3,263	Bran (w/added sugar	
Soy sauce	7,325	and malt extract)	1,060
Herring, smoked	6,231	Knockwurst	1,010
Olives		Spices	
greek style	3,288	chili powder	1,010
green	2,400	parsley	452
Seaweed, raw, kelp	3,007	dill weed	208
dulse	2,085	basil	34
Bacon (canad.), cooked	2,555	paprika	34
Salami	2,260	garlic powder	26
Caviar, granular	2,200	Cornflakes (ready to	1,005
Salad dressing		eat)	826
italian	2,092	Butter, regular	
french	1,370	Milk, cow	526
blue cheese	1,097	powdered skim	118
russian	868	condensed (unsw.)	52
thousand island	700	skim	49
Cheese		whole	
parmesan (grated)	1,862	Eggs	338
blue	1,395	fried	257
provolone	876	scrambled	122
brie	629	hard-cooked	
cheddar	620	Chicken, broiled	
monterey	536	flesh and skin	292
mozzarella	373	Spinach, raw	159
swiss	260	cooked	92
ricotta	84	Ice cream, vanilla	87

Diuretics

Diuretics are a type of medication that has been traditionally used to control high blood pressure through regulation of body fluid balance. This is achieved by an increase in urine output. In a similar fashion, it's thought that these drugs can alter the fluid balance in the inner ear which leads to depletion of endolymph and an improvement of the hydrops. Several studies have shown that salt restriction as a first-line therapy with the addition of diuretic use results in improvement in the symptoms of vertigo experienced in Ménière's disease. Diuretics are considered by many physicians as part of the maintenance therapy for vertigo, which means treatment and prevention between vertigo attacks.

Furthermore, some diuretics, notably acetazolamide (Diamox™), are effective in improving hearing. However, these drugs are not in general able to prevent the long-term hearing deterioration typically seen in Ménière's disease. Thus, it is interesting to note that diuretics tend to reduce the number and severity of vertigo attacks, but do not have any long term effect on hearing.

Another class of diuretics, known as osmotic diuretics, has shown a dramatic, though temporary improvement in hearing in approximately 60 percent of patients with Ménière's disease. Examples of osmotic diuretics include glycerin, mannitol, urea and isosorbide. The effect of these drugs is to withdraw water from the body (see Table 8-3).

Vestibular Suppressants

Diazepam (Valium™) is the main vestibular suppressant and is believed to reduce imbalance by turning on inhibitory signals to the inner ear. It is particularly useful for treating acute attacks of vertigo. The usual dose in Ménière's disease for adults is 5 mg orally every 4 to 6 hours. An initial dose of 5 mg can also be administered intravenously. Diazepam is part of a class of drugs known as benzodiazepines. This drug and others in its class cause sedation, incoordination and paradoxically may cause dizziness. Other rare side effects are

Table 8-3: Diuretics

Name	Class of Drug	Usual Dose	Actions	Adverse Effects
Hydrochlor-thiazide (HCTZ)	Thiazide	50 mg/day + Potassium supplements	Blocks salt reabsorption in kidney; causes water loss by kidney.	Dehydration, Low potassium, Hyperglycemia, High uric acid in blood.
HCTZ+tri-amterine (Dyazide,™ Maxzide™)	Combination of Thiazide and Potassium-sparing diuretics	One tablet/day	Same as HCTZ but potassium is conserved	As with HCTZ but potassium levels are normal
Furosemide (Lasix™)	Potassium-lasting diuretic	10-80 mg/day	Increases volume of urine excreted by kidney	Excessive water loss, low blood pressure, low potassium
Amilioride	Potassium sparing diuretic		Reduces potassium secretion by kidneys but causes salt and water loss	Not a strong diuretic. Can lead to excess potassium retention
Acetazolamide (Diamox™)	Carbonic Anhydrase Inhibitors	250 mg 2x/day or 500 mg timed-release pill once per day	Inhibits sodium bicarbonate re-absorption in kidney causing water loss. Useful for acute attacks of vertigo	Numbness/tingling, GI problems, anorexia, drowsiness/fatigue, transient visual problems, increase the symptoms of gout
Methazolamide (Neptazane™)	Carbonic Anhydrase Inhibitor	50 mg/day – 5 days/week for 3 months	Shown to be effective in controlling symptoms of Ménière's.	Skin rash, headaches, diarrhea

respiratory depression and cardiac arrest which occur more commonly in the elderly and severely ill. This drug should be avoided in those with chronic lung diseases and sleep apnea. Other benzodiazepines of note are Lorazepam (Ativan™) and Alprazolam (Xanax™).

Antiemetics

Table 8-4 lists the drugs commonly prescribed to control nausea that ensues from an attack of vertigo. Antihistamines, anticholinergics, antiserotoninergics and antidopaminergic drugs are included in this group. Anticholinergics, such as scopolamine increase motion tolerance and unlike antihistamines are less effective in treating symptoms after they have already appeared. These drugs have prominent side effects such as dry mouth, dilated pupils and sedation. Antihistamines also prevent motion sickness but are more effective in reducing the severity of symptoms even after their onset.

The choice of agent depends on the route of drug administration and the side effect profile. Oral agents are used for mild nausea. Suppositories are used in those unable to absorb the oral agents due to vomiting, and the injectable forms are used in the emergency room or hospital.

Aminoglycosides

The toxic effects of these antibiotics on the ear are well established. Streptomycin and gentamicin are primarily toxic to the vestibular or balance part of the inner ear. Older established treatments for Ménière's disease included the use of systemic streptomycin injected intramuscularly twice daily for periods of days to weeks in patients with debilitating disease in both ears or one-sided disease in the only hearing ear. Many doctors report control of vertigo in almost all patients when using this treatment. However, many clinicians advocate lower dosages and fewer injections to achieve control of vertigo. Many claim that the treatment of choice for bilateral Ménière's disease is administration of low doses of intramuscular streptomycin.

Table 8-4: Antiemetics *(continued on page 184)*

Name	Class of Drug	Usual Dose	Side Effects	Indicat- ions
Droperidol (Inapsine™)	Neuroleptic	2.5 mg or 5 mg sublin- gual	Sedating, hypoten- sion	Alleviate nausea and vomiting in Ménière's
Granisetron (Kytril™)	5HT3 antag- onist	1 mg by mouth twice a day or 10 micro- grams/kg IV daily	Headache	Useful in treating nau- sea, but expensive and not used as first-line therapy
Meclizine (Antivert,™ Bonine™)	Antihistamine, anticholinergic	12.5-25 mg by mouth every 4-6 hours as needed	Sedating, precau- tions in glaucoma and prostate enlarge- ment	A useful antiemetic to prevent nau- sea and vom- iting due to vestibular disease
Dimenhydri- nate (Dramamine™)	Antihistamine	50 to 100 mg 3-4x/day	Mild drowsiness	Useful in preventing and treating vertigo in Ménière's
Diphenhydramine (Benadryl™)	Antihistamine	50 mg orally as initial dose	Drowsiness	Motion sick- ness, nau- sea, vomit- ing and pre- venting ver- tigo attacks; not typical for acute vertigo
Dronabinol (Marinol™) Delta 9 THL (tetrahydro- cannabinol)	Cannabinoid and sympath- ominetic	2.9, 5.0, 10 mg pills 1-3x/day	Fainting, increased appetite "the wanted effect" abuse potential	Nausea, vom- iting, anorex- ia

Table 8-4 *(continued):* Antiemetics

Name	Class of Drug	Usual Dose	Side Effects	Indica-tions
Metochlopramide (Reglan™)	Dopamine antagonist and stimu-lates the GI tract motili-ty	10 mg by mouth 3x/day or 10 mg intra-muscularly	Restlessnes, drowsiness	Antiemetic that inhibits the brain centers for vomiting
Ondansetron (Zofran™)	5HT3 antag-onist	4-8 mg by mouth 3x/day	Precaution in liver dys-function	As with Kytril
Perphenazine (Trilafon™)	Phenothiazine	2-4 mg by mouth up to 4x/day or 5 mg intra-muscularly 3x/day	Sedating and extrapyra-midal (move-ment) effects	Treating vertigo and motion sick-ness
Prochlorperazine (Compazine™)	Phenothiazine	5 mg 3x/day or 10 mg intramuscu-larly or by mouth every 6-8 hours	Sedating, extrapyra-midal effects	As with Trilafon
Promethazine (Phenergan™)	Phenothiazine	12.5 mg by mouth or intramuscu-larly every 6-8 hours	Sedating, extrapyra-midal effects	As with Trilafon
Trimethobenza mide (Tigan™)	Similar to phenoth-iazines	200 mg intramuscu-larly three times/day	Sedating, extrapyra-midal effects	As with Trilafon

Pressure Chamber Therapy

Pressure chamber therapy involves the use of a decompression chamber that causes a reduction in air pressure and then translates into a relatively positive pressure in the middle ear space. This results in a reduction of the endolymphatic hydrops. It has been noted to be successful in providing long-lasting improvement in both hearing and vertigo in about 45 percent of Ménière's sufferers.

Calcium Channel Blockers

A promising group of drugs in the treatment of vertigo are the calcium channel blockers. These agents, which are among the mainstays of hypertensive therapy, are widely used outside of the U.S. to treat vertigo. Flunarizine and cinnarizine are popular choices and have both anticholinergic and/or anhihistaminic effects. Some drugs in this group such as verapamil have strong constipating effects and thus can manage the diarrhea caused by vestibular imbalance. These drugs can also be effective in Ménière's disease and other forms of vertigo that have a strong association with migraines.

Calcium channel blockers are often very effective in controlling the symptoms of migraine. These drugs have not been approved for the treatment of vertigo in the U.S., but some sources indicate that amelioration (suppression) of vertigo attacks occurs in up to 1/3 of their patients. Nimodopine has been demonstrated effectiveness in the treatment of Ménière's patients who have failed diuretic therapy. Further studies will determine the exact role of these drugs in the management of dizziness and vertigo.

Role of Allergy in the Treatment of Ménière's Disease

The role of allergy as a potential cause of Ménière's disease is strengthened by several observations:

- the onset of symptoms and the ingestion of certain foods

- a seasonal or weather change
- a known history or family history of allergy
- a history of Ménière's symptoms that are either steroid dependent or sensitive
- involvement of both ears with Ménière's disease, and
- failure to respond to the usual traditional medical and surgical treatment of Ménière's disease.

Both inhalant and food allergies have been linked with symptoms of Ménière's disease. Many of the clinical characteristics of Ménière's disease suggest an underlying immune or autoimmune cause (the body's immune system attacking itself). Its propensity to wax and wane and become active again after long periods of remission suggests an inflammatory cause for this disease. It is also bilateral in a significant number of cases and often responsive, at least initially, to steroid treatment. Medical reports have listed the estimate of (bilateral) Ménière's Disease developing in the second ear can occur in 15-70 percent of all patients depending on what criteria is used. Most doctors believe it is probably about 20 percent of patients with Ménière's who will develop it in the other ear at some point in their life to a significant or noticeable degree. It is usually less severe when it affects the other ear. Patients who develop bilateral Ménière's within a short period of time however, tend to have a more stormy course.

Thus, there's a strong suggestion that Ménière's disease is caused or influenced by autoimmune factors, but the most accurate tests currently available to diagnose an autoimmune abnormality are usually normal. Therefore, we might wonder whether there are other immune causes for the development of the symptoms.

Food allergies are increasingly being recognized as an important cause of the symptoms of Ménière's disease. The propensity to develop a food allergy, as well as inhalant allergy, is inherited. Indications of a possible food allergy include craving or addiction to a particular food, perennial symptoms, a history of infantile allergy to foods producing symptoms such as frequent croup, eczema, colic, excess fluid retention and improved symptoms after a fast.

Food allergies can be clinically divided into two types: cyclic and fixed. "Cyclic food allergies" occur several hours after ingesting the offending food. This is the most common among food allergies and constitutes approximately 95 percent of food hypersensitivities. Symptoms vary depending on the quantity of food ingested. "Fixed food allergies" are not exposure dependent; eating the offending food will produce symptoms either immediately or after a certain time.

To establish a diagnosis of food allergy, the best test is the oral challenge feeding test. This test can determine a cause and effect relationship between ingestion of a given food and the production of symptoms. Food allergies can also be diagnosed from a clinical standpoint by the subcutaneous or intradermal provocative food test. The provocative food test has been shown to correlate well with the results of oral challenge food testing.

Food allergies are best treated by eliminating the offending food(s) from the diet in all forms until clinical improvement appears, eventually followed by the development of limited immune tolerance. This point is usually achieved in an adult after three months of dietary avoidance and is determined by a deliberate challenge feeding test. If no symptoms are produced a person may reintroduce the food back into the diet.

A very small percentage of patients have a fixed reaction to the food which persists despite the dietary avoidance. Sometimes, if there are multiple food allergens or you're unable to avoid eating the food, treatment by injection or sublingual drops of the neutralizing dose established by provocative food testing will provide clinical improvement.

The best treatment for inhalant allergies is avoidance of the offending allergen. However, rarely is only one significant allergen the culprit and for patients sensitive to multiple allergens, avoidance is rarely sufficient to control symptoms. Pharmacotherapy, immunotherapy or both may be necessary for relief.

A recommended treatment regimen for Ménière's disease has been promoted by the House Ear Institute in Los Angeles, CA. This entails an attempt to suppress the vestibular symptoms and treat the endolymphatic hydrops. For the treatment of acute vertigo, oral diazepam is recommended as it controls the symptoms of nausea, vomiting and vertigo seen in the majority of Ménière's patients. In cases that do not respond, meclizine 25 to 100 mg orally, dimenhydrinate 50 mg orally or intramuscularly, hyoscine 0.6 mg subcutaneously, droperidol 5 mg intravenously, or diazepam 5 to 20 mg slow intravenously may be warranted.

Maintenance therapy involves preventing acute vertigo attacks. This is accomplished by diet control and the use of diuretics. A typical starting regimen of diuretics is 50 mg of Hydrochlorthiazide (see Table 8-3) supplemented with potassium daily or Dyazide™, one tablet per day. If the diuretics are not effective, then vasodilators may be considered. The role of many of these medications, such as histamine and betahistine to improve blood flow to the inner ear, though temporarily relieving vertigo in many patients, has still not been defined adequately.

Antioxidants and Dizziness

Antioxidants help to counteract the harmful effects of damaging ROS (reactive oxygen species) which are oxygen radicals produced by our bodies during the process of energy production. The body has a host of enzymes that protect us from these harmful radicals, but unfortunately these diminish with age. Antioxidants have been implicated in many disorders in which balance is affected. For example, in Ménière's disease antioxidants may accumulate due to injuries within the endolymphatic sac from changing fluid balance or possible immune system reactions.

In order to buffer our bodies, oral supplementation with antioxidants and vitamins has been advocated by many leading authorities.

Herbals in the Treatment of Vertigo

There are several herbs that may be beneficial if you suffer with severe imbalance or vertigo. Table 8-5 lists some of the more well-known herbs and their properties. If you are to consider any, discuss them with your physician.

Vitamins and Minerals*

There are some specific nutrients that have been popularized to treat vertigo. Some include:

- Magnesium (Grain, nuts, beans, green vegetables and bananas)
- Calcium (Yogurt, milk and cheese)
- Potassium (Fresh fruits and vegetables)
- Lipoflavinoids
- B vitamins
- Multivitamin supplements
- Antioxidant supplements

Betahistine*

Betahistine hydrochloride (Serc™) is in the histamine family. Histamines are inflammatory molecules released from tissue injury. For example, allergy sufferers release excessive histamine when exposed to certain environmental irritants. Antihistamines are taken to control allergic reactions. These have received considerable attention in the past few years. It has an interesting mechanism of action. It stimulates H1 and H2 (histamine) receptors and has strong H3 antagonist activity. It's paradoxical that both blockade and stimulation of H1 receptors results in an anti-vertigo effect. This is clinically realized with histamine which has a positive effect on dizziness (activates H1 and H2 receptors) while flunarizine and cinnarizine which are H1 receptor antagonists also improve dizziness.

*There are no evidence-based medical studies that have demonstrated its effectiveness in controlling vertigo.

Table 8-5: Herbs Used To Treat Dizziness And Vertigo

Name	Claims	Actions	Contraindica-tions	Side Effects	Interactions
Ginkgo biloba	Improves circulation. Treats Alzheimer's, Other cognitive disorders, tinnitus, vertigo	Vasodilator, adaptogen, stimulant, antioxidant	Careful in patients taking anticoagulants, such as warfarin (Coumadin™)	Rare GI upset (seen with off brands)	Coumadin heparin, other anticoagulants. No significant interaction with aspirin
Ginger (Zingiber officinale)	Alleviates nausea, dyspepsia, vomiting and motion sickness	Antiemetic, antispasmodic, anti-inflammatory & hypo-glycemic activity	Same as for Gingko biloba. May lower blood glucose levels which can be an unwanted effect particularly in patients with pre-existing hypoglycemia.	Heartburn, in large doses on empty stomach	Same as for Gingko biloba

Ginseng (panax ginseng)	Fatigue, depression, stress, general well being, sexual energy and digestion	Adaptogenic (and promotes secretion of ACTH-causing release of endorphins and enkephelins) stimulant, lowers RBS, inhibits platelet aggregation	Avoid in patient with hypertension and diabetes mellitus and in pregnancy; may interfere with anticoagulant therapy	In high doses can cause insomnia, anxiety, GI upset	Do not use with other anticoagulants or stimulants (ie. caffeine), MAOI's, antipsychotics
Blessed thistle (cnicus benedictus)	Stimulates appetite, digestion, relieves dyspepsia, treats upper respiratory infections, antibacterial	Galactagogue-stimulates lactation	None noted	Large doses-GI upset or immune suppression	Sensitization to mugwort & cornflower. Can increase stomach acid therefore interfering with antacids

Table 8-5 *(continued)*: Herbs Used To Treat Dizziness And Vertigo.

Name	Claims	Actions	Contraindica-tions	Side Effects	Interactions
Hawthorn berry (crataegus oxycanthus)	Treats athero-sclerosis, arrhythmia, hypertension & improves car-diac output & coronary blood flowTreats ath-erosclerosis, arrhythmia, hypertension & improves car-diac output & coronary blood flow	Cardiac and sedative	Do not use with other car-diac drugs (digoxin, anti-hypertensive therapy)	Mildly sedative	Avoid digitalis or foxglove
Gotu kola (centella asi-atica)	Improves mem-ory, treats hypothyroidism	Restorative, stops bleeding and promotes wound healing	None noted	None noted (rarely may cause skin irri-tation)	Can lead to increase in blood glucose, cholesterol, triglycerides

Cocculus compositum (vertigoheel)	Treat anxiety, nervousness, chronic tinnitus, vertigo	Improves brain blood flow	None noted	In high doses: headache, dizziness, nausea & vomiting, sleepiness, tonic-clonic spasms	Avoid treating with other GABA-ergic agents
Black cohosh (Cimicifuga racemosa)	Treat anxiety, nervousness, chronic tinnitus, vertigo	Improves brain blood flow	None noted	In high doses: nausea, vomiting, dizziness	None noted
Ligustrum (Ligustrum Lucidum)	Treats tinnitus, dizziness, back pain	Enhances blood flow, anti-allergic, anti-inflammatory	None noted	None noted	None noted
Valerian Root (Valeriana Officinalis)	Promotes sleep, improves dizziness	Inhibition of brain pathways involved in anxiety and vertigo	None noted	Drowsiness. Cardiac complications in high doses (530 mg-2g up to 5x/day)	Avoid if taking anti-anxiety meds. Do not take if operating machinery

Table 8-5 *(continued)*: Herbs Used To Treat Dizziness And Vertigo.

Name	Claims	Actions	Contraindica-tions	Side Effects	Interactions
Kava Kava (Piper Methysticum)	Treats anxiety, stress, insomnia. In high doses: acts as a hypnotic, muscle relaxant	Similar to Benzodiazapenes	Should not be used in patients with endogenous depression or during pregnancy/lactation. Additionally, it should not be used for more than 3 months continuously without medical advice	Drowsiness, balance disturbances & mild GI upset. Concern about liver toxicity/failure even in normal doses	Should not be taken concomitantly with CNS depressants such as alcohol, benzodiazepines or antipsychotics

Since betahistine is a weak H1 receptor agonist, its effect is likely mediated through some other mechanism, perhaps through the antagonism of H3 receptors. Nonetheless, it is widely accepted that the primary mechanism of action appears to be linked to increased blood flow to the inner ear.

An elegant and critical review of the literature has been completed by Schmidt in 1992.[2] The reader is referred to this article for details. Although Serc™ is not FDA approved for commercial distribution in the U.S., it is permitted for compounding pharmacies to make it with a doctor's prescription. It has had mixed success in the management of balance disorders in Europe and Canada. It is primarily indicated for Ménière's disease in a dosage of 8-16 mg three times per day, but has been used for many types of dizziness. Most people report a positive effect within a few days (if there is one), but it seems to be moderately effective in suppressing the symptoms of Ménière's disease. You should work closely with your physician on establishing the particular dosage for yourself. Common side effects are facial flushing and headache. If you experience these, your dosage should be reduced.

Other Alternatives for Vertigo

In addition to herbal and nutritional strategies, patients with balance disturbances have experienced improvement in their symptoms using a variety of complementary and integrative medicine practices. These include acupuncture, osteopathic and chiropractic manipulation, cranial sacral therapy, St. John's neuromuscular therapy, T'ai Chi, biofeedback, meditation and relaxation therapy, to name a few.

Acupuncture, which involves the insertion and manipulation of needles at numerous points in the body, has been used to treat disorders of balance. Ironically, traditional Chinese medicine focuses on keeping the "balance" between two opposing yet complementary natural forces: the "yin" and the "yang." The *yin* force signifies peace and tranquility and represents darkness and coldness. The *yang* force is depicted as aggressive and represents light and heat. Although the primary use of acupuncture has been for pain relief, its application in treating disorders of balance has been described in the medical literature. This therapy is one of the most studied alternative medical practices. Studies have shown positive results in the treatment of a variety of conditions.

Cranio-sacral therapy is a type of holistic therapy that uses touch to diagnose and treat the cranio-sacral system. This system refers to the skull, spinal column and the supporting structures, such as the cerebrospinal fluid that protect the brain and spinal cord. Using a very light touch, the practitioner attempts to feel the cranial rhythmic impulse (CRI) of the cerebrospinal fluid. The goal of the treatment is to restore the fluid balance by allowing free movement of the CRI. This contributes to self-healing and the restoration of function. A session normally lasts about 30 to 60 minutes and is aimed at disorders of many systems, including those involved in balance.

There are many other complementary/alternative therapeutic options for the management of dizziness which go well beyond the scope of this book. The reader is encouraged to be receptive of complementary and integrative medicine options, but to remain objectively critical of unapproved therapeutic modalities. Our goal must be to enhance the wellness and promote the health of our patients. Sometimes this requires extending the scope and considering alternatives when conventional options have been less than successful.

Proven therapeutic options should be discussed in association with viable complementary/integrative medicine (CIM) strategies. If a reasonable alternative option exists, it may be prudent to consider its use. Patients often have the misconception that "natural" means safe. This is truly a fallacy and one perpetuated by inappropriate advertising. Quality control and standardization is important to consider. The only enforceable law regarding quality control stems from the Dietary and Supplement Health and Education Act of 1994 (DSHEA) which places the burden of labeling claims and label information on the manufacturer. Since there is no independent oversight of this industry there's always the potential for problems. It is these contributors' opinion that risks are relatively low. Patients should always consider consulting with their doctor before taking any complementary treatments. Some of these can contain potent medications or cause side effects.

Clearly, there are some products that appear to be less effective and have a higher degree of patient sensitivity reactions than others. Two examples are with Ginkgo biloba and Echinacea products. When discussing this with patients, the senior author informs them that the Ginkgo bottle must say either 24 percent ginkgo-flavonoids, 24 percent ginkgoglycosides or 50:1 standardized extract. Echinacea poses a particular problem in that there are at least nine different subtypes known, ie. E. purpurea, E. pallida and E. angustofolia. The German Commission E rates herbs as positive or negative. E. angustofolia is rated as a negative herb (not because of harm, but because of lack of an effect) whereas E. purpurea leaf and pallida root have been shown to be effective at enhancing T and B cell function. Interestingly, most health food stores sell E. angustofolia; the subtype that has been shown to have little or no immune enhancing effects. Thus, it is incumbent upon the physician or pharmacist to begin to have an understanding of the subtleties in the realm of CIM. It is also important to realize that herbal/nutritional-pharmaceutical interactions occur, there is an increasing amount of information becoming available on the subject. Lastly, we should ask these questions of CIM or even traditional medicine:

- What disease or condition is being treated?
- What is the conventional therapy?
- What are the CIM therapeutic options?
- What is the benefit to the patient from conventional therapy and from CIM therapy?
- What are the risks of conventional or CIM therapies?
- What is the cost?
- Does it work?

It's becoming increasingly evident that collaboration between physicians and complementary and alternative medicine practitioners is needed to tackle the problem of dizziness, since there are so many causes, yet so few established treatment regimens. It may very well be the best scenario for patient care, patient satisfaction and possibly even cost containment. We can no longer ignore the masses. CIM is not a trend. It is being implemented widely and we have an obligation to our patients and to ourselves to study and learn about the alternatives and put an end to the ones that don't work, embracing the ones that do.

The medical management of vertigo and dizziness is a formidable challenge, largely because we don't know the precise reasons for what triggers them. A positive point is that medical (not surgical) treatment is the primary mode of therapy. In fact, 80 percent of Ménière's disease patients are treated effectively with non-surgical therapies. It's not clear why these balance disturbances occur and equally elusive is how the drugs work to remedy the problem. Thus, it's crucially important that a good doctor-patient relationship be created and that you work together to find the most appropriate therapy, tailoring it to your specific situation.

Following an initial attack, a person is often extremely apprehensive and requires considerable support and reassurance. Psychological support is often the most important aspect of medical management. This should include an explanation of the cause of dizziness/vertigo, the way the disease usually progresses and the different types of treatment to address the problem. For example, although there are no cures for Ménière's disease, it is important to note that the symptoms can be well managed with a combination of therapies described previously. With the help of your physician an appropriate regimen can be tailored to this end.

Bibliography

U.S. Department of Agriculture. Composition of Foods, Agriculture Handbook Series No. 8. Washington DC: Agriculture Research Services, 1980.

Schmidt JT and Huizing EH. The clinical drug trial in Ménière's disease with emphasis on the effect of betahistine SR. Acta Otolaryngol Suppl. 1992;497:1-189.

CHAPTER NINE

Surgical Treatment

Dennis Poe, MD
Department of Otology and Laryngology
Harvard Medical School, Children's Hospital of Boston
Massachusetts Eye and Ear Infirmary
Boston, Massachusetts

Dr. Poe earned his MD from SUNY Syracuse, his residency in otolaryngology-head and neck surgery at the University of Chicago, and a subspecialty fellowship in neurotology with the Otology Group in Nashville, Tennessee. He is a full-time faculty member in the department of Otology and Laryngology, Harvard Medical School and Children's Hospital of Boston. He is also on staff at the Massachusetts Eye and Ear Infirmary. He has published a number of scientific research articles and patient information writings on medical and surgical treatments for Meniere's disease. He has done pioneering work in minimally invasive surgery of the ear.

Making Decisions
About Surgery and Procedures for Vertigo

Most people with vertigo will be able to adequately control the condition through conservative medical treatments. There is a small percentage of patients in whom medical therapy will not sufficiently control their attacks of vertigo and for whom surgical options will be considered. Surgery and office procedures are invasive in nature. Anything invasive generally has the potential for more side effects or risks compared to medical treatments. It's natural that you and your doctor will want to exhaust all possible medical treatments for your condition before considering surgical options.

Surgery is intended only for the forms of inner ear disorders that cause repeated attacks, spells or paroxysms (intense attacks) of vertigo. Frequent attacks of vertigo may lead to chronic disequilibrium. If the attacks can be stopped, then the brain and vestibular system have a chance to recover and compensate over time, hopefully leading to resolution of the disequilibrium. Patients with chronic disequilibrium, but no active vertigo attacks, have a compensation problem that won't be helped by surgery. In fact, surgery could worsen their chronic compensation difficulties by altering the status of the balance system and adding to the disequilibrium.

When the inner ear is subjected to intermittent irritation or injury, it will result in an acute disturbance in your balance. This disrupts the vestibular nerve outputs from the affected inner ear and puts it into conflict with the information being received by the brain from the other normal inner ear. This conflict in information is confusing to the brain and causes a profound disturbance in the vestibular system that we perceive as vertigo. Once the attack of vertigo ceases, you may feel immediately back to normal if the spell was brief or mild. You may also feel quite a lot of imbalance or disequilibrium for minutes, hours, days or even weeks after such an event. The length of time it takes to recover your balance after a vertigo attack depends on how severely it may affect your inner ear, how much permanent damage done may occur, and how well you tend to compensate.

Your balance is maintained by the brain coordinating inputs from the vestibular systems of both inner ears, your vision, and your sensation of position and touch in your legs (proprioception). Your compensatory abilities depend on the remaining elements of your balance to cover up the weakness in your one balance nerve. If you're in good condition and exercise regularly, your compensation abilities will be better than someone inactive, elderly, or with problems involving vision and proprioception.

Each time a vertigo attack occurs it's as though a monkey wrench has just been thrown into your balance machinery. The amount of damage done by the monkey wrench determines how quickly you can regain your balance. This process can be expected to take some time. Exercising and working on your balance can speed your recovery. I always emphasize to patients how important it is to understand that you can have a great deal of influence over how quickly you can get over vertigo attacks. Exercising will not help prevent the attacks. This is where you depend on medical or surgical treatment. The medical and surgical treatment is designed to minimize or stop the balance attacks or "monkey wrenches" into the machinery and has been previously presented and discussed. If the balance attacks occur frequently, you may never have enough time between attacks to regain full control of your balance or be free of disequilibrium.

Patients with frequent vertigo attacks can therefore have chronic imbalance or disequilibrium and they often feel that they have developed a new condition. In fact, the condition itself has not fundamentally changed; it is only that the vertigo attacks have become so frequent you never have a chance to recover from them completely. Most patients with a vertigo attack once a month or less will have periods of time where their balance can seem normal. When spells occur more than once a month the secondary disequilibrium can become chronic. This is roughly the break point at which many patients decide they can no longer tolerate their vertigo condition and need to pursue more aggressive treatment by undergoing some type of surgical procedure.

Most of the surgery for vertigo is done for Ménière's disease, a condition in which the episodes of dizziness can be quite disabling and occur unexpectedly. Good medical control of Ménière's disease is felt to be one or two clusters of episodes per year during which time there's an increase of fluid pressure inside the ear (endolymphatic hydrops). While the pressure is high you could experience one or more attacks within a one to two week period after which the condition will typically improve. One or two clusters of attacks per year would be considered reasonable medical control. Most patients, of course, do not like the thought of experiencing these vertigo attacks and subsequent disequilibrium. It may even cost them a few days of work, but most people feel they can handle episodes limited to a couple times a year and generally prefer not to undergo a surgical procedure. When the condition occurs more than once monthly, most people seriously consider a surgical procedure.

Benign paroxysmal positional vertigo (BPPV) usually causes less severe vertigo attacks than Ménière's disease and is sometimes treated by surgery. Vertigo attacks due to BPPV may range from mild to severe and generally do not last any more than about a minute, but can recur by repeating the head movements that precipitate the vertigo. Many people will experience this vertigo and have no disequilibrium afterwards, but some will have particularly strong positional vertigo followed by some imbalance or disequilibrium for minutes or even hours later.

When vertigo spells or attacks become so frequent that there's chronic imbalance and disequilibrium, it's important to understand that surgery will not automatically stop the chronic disequilibrium. Surgical treatment is designed to stop the vertigo attacks—that is, stop the "monkey wrenches" from being thrown into the machinery. It may then take some time to repair the machinery. Once the vertigo attacks stop, your body has achieved a state in which it can make some repairs that will not be disrupted by another "monkey wrench." Exercises for your balance such as those discussed in Chapter 10 (on vestibular rehabilitation) will be the principle means of overcoming the disequilibrium following surgery.

It is also possible that certain types of surgery such as labyrinthectomy or chemical labyrinthectomy (gentamicin injections into the ear) or vestibular nerve section to cut the vestibular nerve may make your balance considerably worse before you get better. These so called destructive operations are in effect destroying most or all of your remaining vestibular nerve on the affected side. This means that when your inner ear undergoes another vertigo attack and a "monkey wrench" is once again thrown into the balance machinery, the vestibular nerve has been disabled so that the signals of a disturbance will not be able to reach the brain.

This is one instance in which if your brain doesn't know about it, it can't hurt you. The brain will not perceive any alteration in its information and will continue to receive only the normal inputs from your good side. You'll therefore not experience a vertigo attack even when there may be active hydrops in the remaining portion of the inner ear. Once you are free from the vertigo attacks, then the process of vestibular compensation can begin as your brain relearns to coordinate the inputs from one vestibular organ, vision, and your sense of position and touch in the legs (proprioception).

Your equilibrium depends on inputs from three systems: your vestibular system, vision, and proprioception. These are coordinated in the brain at all times. These systems are also redundant whereby injury to any one of these three systems will not cause a fundamental disturbance in your balance. If you have problems with two of the three systems, however, you will begin to experience significant balance problems. If you have a vestibular disorder and then add a visual problem or proprioception problem, you can expect to have significant vestibular compensation difficulties. Visual problems could include cataracts, retinal detachment, macular degeneration, change of glasses, and so forth. The most common proprioception problems would be peripheral neuropathy in legs due to diabetes, back problems and other neurological conditions. A failure of any two of these three systems will give you significant problems with vestibular compensation.

What to Expect from Medical Therapy

So what is the goal of medical therapy for dizziness problems? Certainly for lightheadedness due to general medical conditions such as cardiac, vascular and metabolic disorders, the goal is to identify the underlying medical problem(s) and treat them appropriately. Vestibular problems are treated with medications and physical therapy when appropriate.

There are three strategies for conservative management of vestibular disorders:

1. Use of medication to prevent vertigo attacks by treatment of any underlying condition.

2. Suppression of existing vertigo or chronic disequilibrium symptoms with medications.

3. Efforts to improve vestibular compensation, usually through vestibular rehabilitation.

It's important to remember these three different types of treatment when trying to understand the goals of your medical therapy and what role surgery may play in the event of medical failure.

Common vertigo conditions in which the underlying condition can be treated are Ménière's disease, benign paroxysmal positional vertigo, and vestibular migraines.

Low sodium dietary restrictions are recommended as the most important treatment for Ménière's disease (see the Low Sodium Table in Chapter 8, page 179). The body uses sodium to regulate fluid pressure which is why patients with high blood pressure are placed on low sodium diets. Similarly, diuretics or water pills are used to some degree to aid in reducing the body's content of sodium. Reduction of stress and potent stimulants such as caffeine and nicotine can be helpful. In this way we try to control the spells as much as possible, minimizing the frequency and severity of vertigo attacks.

Ménière's disease typically runs a course of several years and then may eventually "burn itself out." The average time it may take for the condition to go away on its own is approximately ten years but statistics for this show a very wide bell-shaped curve centered over a ten year average. This means that many people can have Ménière's lasting for a shorter period and an equally large number can have Ménière's exceeding the ten years. We can't predict in any individual how long you will suffer with Ménière's disease. Our efforts are directed at trying to control the episodes as much as possible. We generally consider someone under good control who has episodes of fluid swelling (hydrops) in the ear and vertigo spells over a one to two week period occurring once or twice a year. Each episode of hydrops may cause a little bit of cumulative damage to the inner ear so it is hoped that the hearing and vestibular systems will be injured as little as possible throughout the individual's course of their Ménière's disease. When the episodes of vertigo are as rare as a few times a year,

disequilibrium following the spells should be minimally troublesome as well. We consider a patient in remission when
they have had no attacks or spells of vertigo for two years.

The Use of Medications in Ménière's Disease And Other Vestibular Disorders

Vestibular suppressants (tranquilizers and antihistamines) sedate the central nervous system and balance system
to reduce dizziness symptoms. <u>They do not physically improve
your balance</u> but you will feel a reduction in spinning vertigo
and imbalance with movements. They can reduce nausea and
vomiting. If you are unfortunate enough to have a severe
attack of vertigo requiring you to go to an emergency room,
they are very likely to pump you full of intravenous vestibular suppressants such as diazepam even to the point where
you may have to sleep off the after effects for several hours.
Sleeping peacefully definitely beats spinning vertigo, nausea,
and vomiting.

Doctors usually recommend vestibular suppressants for
symptom relief on an "as needed basis," referred to as "prn" in
medical lingo. Think of taking these medications in the same
way that you would take aspirin to help relieve a headache.
You wouldn't even think of taking aspirin on a daily basis for
the rest of your life just to prevent headaches for the rest of
your life. Unfortunately, vertigo is such a disturbing symptom
that once people have experienced it, they will often take
these sedating vestibular suppressants round-the-clock for
weeks, months, or even indefinitely, fearing that if they stop
the symptoms might recur. <u>Vestibular suppressants are not
preventive medications</u>; they only reduce the symptoms. They
will not prevent your next vertigo attack! If you're having a
lot of attacks of vertigo, it may make sense to take medication
round-the-clock or on a daily basis to reduce the symptoms at
a time when spells are coming hard and fast. If you're having
a lot of vertigo attacks, you'd be expected to have a lot of secondary dysequilibrium and chronic medication could help
until you feel start feeling better.

There can be a strong placebo effect in the use of medications that should not be underestimated. A doctor close to me once asked me to write her a prescription for a scopolamine (antiemetic) patch so that she could go on a boat trip that day. She used it and returned that afternoon joyously singing the medication's praises that she'd never been able to enjoy a small boat ride before without getting dreadfully motion sick. As she literally jumped for joy the patch suddenly fell from behind her ear, right in front of my eyes! I wondered how the adhesive could have given away like that and examined the patch only to find that the protective plastic barrier was still intact and the sticky medicated surface had never been exposed. The patch couldn't have worked because only the plastic barrier had been placed against her skin and miraculously had held up all day without falling off earlier. Both of us learned a powerful lesson about mind control that day.

The Role of Vestibular Rehabilitation

Vertigo attacks are best controlled by prevention through treatment of the underlying problem. If attacks cannot be prevented, then vestibular suppressants are used to try and suppress them. If they are difficult to suppress, antiemetic medications are added. If the attacks are so frequent that chronic disequilibrium symptoms are present, then some degree of chronic vestibular suppression medication may be used. If vertigo spells cease but chronic disequilibrium persists, then vestibular rehab (rehabilitation) may be recommended.

Vestibular rehab can be as simple as participating in active exercises such as walking, jogging, swimming or any sport involving chasing a ball, generally performing any movements that stimulate your balance. Stationary exercises such as weight lifting, bicycling and Nordic tracks are great cardiovascular training, but really do very little for your balance. In order to best stimulate all three aspects of your balance system (vestibular system, vision, and proprioception), it's best to perform some form of exercise where you are moving from point A to point B under your own two feet as opposed to a stationary bicycle or treadmill. Formal physical therapy for rehab may be recommended when you stop making improvements when exercising on your own.

Medical Treatment for Benign Paroxysmal Positional Vertigo

BPPV is another form of vestibular dysfunction in which treatment of the underlying cause may be possible. Various canalith-repositioning maneuvers discussed in Chapter 6, habituation exercises, and vestibular rehabilitation are done to treat the underlying problem. Vestibular suppressants may be useful when symptoms occur frequently. Antiemetics are rarely used for this condition because the spells subside so quickly that significant nausea is not usually a problem.

Medical Treatment of Vestibular Migraines

Vertigo attacks caused by migraines (see Chapter 4) are treated with medications and dietary restrictions in order to minimize or stop the underlying migraines. Once the vertigo attacks stop, any residual secondary disequilibrium can be helped with exercising or vestibular rehabilitation. Vestibular suppressants and antiemetics are commonly used for vestibular migraines that are not controlled since the vertigo and nausea can be quite severe.

How Surgery Can Help

So what happens if the vertigo spells cannot be controlled? This is the time that surgical options may be introduced. Migraines cannot be treated with surgery and can only be treated with medication and observation of appropriate dietary restrictions. Inner ear disorders that cause vertigo attacks may respond to different types of procedures designed to eliminate the vertigo attacks. It's important to note that surgical procedures do not eliminate the disequilibrium. They are designed to stop the attacks so that your body can subsequently initiate the compensation process. As long as vertigo attacks disrupt your balance system, you're in an unsteady state and you're subject to disequilibrium. If you can stop the vertigo attacks by whatever means necessary, then you have achieved a steady state in your balance system and effective vestibular compensation can begin. Your brain will reorganize how it processes information between the three systems important to your balance (vestibular, vision, proprioception).

Surgery for vertigo is divided into two basic categories: destructive and nondestructive. These will be presented and discussed next. (You may wish to refer to the anatomical parts represented in Figure 5-1 in Chapter 5 on page 116.)

Destructive Procedures

Destructive procedures are intended to destroy most or all the remaining balance organ or balance nerve from a diseased inner ear. When an inner ear is diseased, it causes vertigo whenever it acts up. It doesn't matter whether the injury is caused by a Ménière's attack of hydrops, free floating canalith particles of BPPV bouncing around the semicircular canal, or a perilymphatic fistula.

All unstable inner ear disorders cause waves of abnormal balance signals to race to your brain and compete with the normal balance signals coming from the other inner ear. This conflict in information can provoke a vertigo attack. If the inner ear is surgically or chemically destroyed, or the balance nerve that carries signals from the diseased inner ear to the brain is severed, then abnormal signals cannot reach the brain and you will not have vertigo attacks. If you've been suffering from disequilibrium, your inner ear has achieved a steady state of little to no function. Your brain and all of the systems that play into your balance now have a chance to work positively in restoring your equilibrium.

Destructive procedures include labyrinthectomy, vestibular nerve section and chemical labyrinthectomy.

Labyrinthectomy

Labyrinthectomy is an operation that can be done as a short procedure through the ear canal or as a larger operation making an incision behind the ear and opening up the air-filled sinus called the mastoid. Both operations work quite well. The through-the-ear canal procedure (transcanal labyrinthectomy) does not physically remove the entire inner ear organ and therefore has a greater chance for some recurrence of vertigo in the future. For this reason the transmastoid approach is more commonly used because the surgeon can visibly see all five sensory endings of the vestibular endorgan. Recurrence of vertigo is very unlikely.

Of any operation we do, labyrinthectomy gives you the highest possible success rate for eliminating vertigo attacks. For this reason it's called the "gold standard." However, it's not commonly used because removing the vestibular organ also causes complete deafness in the operated ear since the inner ear hearing organ (the cochlea) is directly connected to the vestibular organ. Losing one's hearing can also result in the brain creating disturbing ringing noises in the ear (tinnitus), but this is fortunately an uncommon side effect of the operation. The operation is favored when there is already little or no useful hearing in the affected ear. We define "useful" hearing as sufficiently good that you could use a hearing aid if desired. When hearing in the affected ear is not "useful," labyrinthectomy may be an appropriate operation for you.

The operation may produce prolonged disequilibrium following the procedure and initially even some vertigo. By cutting out the remaining vestibular organ or nerve the surgeon has suddenly changed the vestibular outputs on that side and the brain will interpret this as yet another vertigo attack that can be as bad as the vertigo attacks you already get, if not worse. The amount of vertigo you experience will depend on how much vestibular function still exists in your inner ear. If the inner ear is already almost dead, cutting out the remaining inner ear function will really not affect you very much. If there is a lot of function in the inner ear, you may have a tremendous amount of vertigo with spinning just as if you were having one of your worst vertigo attacks. So fortunately, you will be in the hospital where you can get intravenous medications to relieve your symptoms.

Generally, spinning vertigo after these operations lasts for a day or two after which you can go home. The vestibular compensation process begins immediately with active walking and head turning exercises to stimulate your balance system. Your vestibular recovery will depend a great deal on how aggressive you are about forcing yourself to walk and making yourself dizzy even though it doesn't feel good to do so. The more aggressive you are about forcing yourself to walk and make yourself dizzy, the faster you'll get over these symptoms. As everyone with vertigo has learned, vertigo and disequilibrium consume a tremendous amount of your energy, so fatigue is a common complaint after such surgery.

Generally, the balance will slowly improve over the next few weeks. Most young patients will resume work in four to six weeks after a labyrinthectomy and are often able to drive a car about that time. Older patients may be looking at six to eight weeks for a reasonable recovery. Bear in mind that you don't magically get better at the six-week mark, but this is a gradual process. When people do resume work they're generally very fatigued by the end of the day. You already know that the more fatigued you are, the more your disequilibrium affects you by the end of the day. It may take an additional several weeks or even months before you feel completely whole again and back to your normal energy levels.

Most patients will feel that they do make a true full recovery. You may notice some degree of disequilibrium if you turn your head very quickly, particularly in the direction of the affected ear. You may also notice some instability with eyes closed or in the dark. Elderly patients may have much more difficulty with their balance recovery and may never completely compensate. Occasionally we see someone who becomes so severely affected that they require the use of a cane or walker after such an operation, but this is generally very elderly patients or those with other neurological problems. Even professional athletes who have undergone this operation have told me that they may have lost some of the razor edge that helped them compete in their sport, but they are still very competitive.

Vestibular Nerve Section

Vestibular nerve section is a neurosurgical approach to cut the vestibular nerve between the brainstem and the inner ear. This is a bigger operation with more risks than a labyrinthectomy. The reason for undergoing a bigger operation is that your balance nerve can be cut, but you can retain your hearing. The hearing and balance nerves (that is, the cochlear and vestibular divisions of the eighth cranial nerve) can be surgically separated close to the brainstem. The vestibular nerve is divided while saving the cochlear nerve and hearing. Although hearing loss can be a complication of the operation, the statistics for hearing preservation are quite good in experienced hands. Instead of one or two days in the hospital as with labyrinthectomy, vestibular nerve section patients are generally in the hospital for two or three days. There is the added side-effect of headache, but it's usually much better than patients expect. Post-operative vertigo and prolonged balance recovery are identical to a labyrinthectomy operation. Therefore, the main reason for choosing this operation is to try to get the highest possible success rate for stopping your vertigo attacks, but also trying to spare your hearing.

Chemical Labyrinthectomy

Chemical labyrinthectomy most commonly today means doing a procedure called intratympanic injection of gentamicin. Intratympanic refers to injection of a medication through the eardrum or tympanic membrane and into your middle ear. The middle ear is the air-filled space behind the drum that can block up on airplanes. Gentamicin is an antibiotic that has the special properties of being toxic to your inner ear, but more toxic to the vestibular organ than to the cochlear or hearing organ. We use this vestibular toxic medication to try to destroy as much of the inner ear balance as possible.

This is a relatively new procedure and there are still many different protocols being used. The most common protocol involves injection of gentamicin into the middle ear and allowing it to stay in place while you lie on your back with your ear turned upward so that the medication will stay against your inner ear for anywhere from 30 to 60 minutes. The procedure is usually repeated one week later. The intent is to remove as much of the balance nerve function as possible without over-shooting and damaging the hearing.

It is an office procedure as opposed to the others which are done usually under general anesthesia. It has a moderate success rate for eliminating vertigo spells that is not quite as high as the labyrinthectomy or vestibular nerve section procedures. Most medical reports showed the operation to be judged successful in improving about 85 percent of the cases as opposed to the other procedures that completely stop the vertigo attacks in generally the mid-ninety percentile range.

Gentamicin toxicity occurs over several days, so the disequilibrium that results from the procedure is spread out over time and is usually not nearly as severe as it is with the other destructive operations. Most patients notice no side effects at all from the first injection. Most will experience the onset of significant disequilibrium about two to four days after the second injection. These symptoms are generally much milder than with the other destructive procedures and most people can continue working throughout this vestibular compensation phase. The disequilibrium subsides with active people after about two to three weeks. There is about a 25 percent chance that you may require a "booster shot" or two in the ear one to two years later as the vestibular organ appears to have some ability to recover some function over time.

The rate of hearing loss is somewhat higher with the intratympanic treatments. Most series using the *titration method* (giving only enough gentamicin to induce disequilibrium) causes deafness in the affected ear in approximately three percent of patients treated. We define deafness as complete hearing loss in the affected ear, unable to use a hearing aid. Twenty-five to forty percent of patients may experience some hearing loss just in the very high frequencies. Most patients treated with gentamicin have Ménière's disease and hearing loss so they'll usually not notice a small amount of additional hearing loss. Patients with normal hearing should be aware that even a small amount of new hearing loss could be very troublesome to them and they may wish to avoid gentamicin. Earlier methods in which fixed standard doses of gentamicin were given in order to completely eliminate all vestibular function had very high deafness rates in the treated ear of 10-25 percent. Patients do not lose hearing in their non-treated ear when they receive intratympanic gentamicin.

Ménière's Disease in Both Ears

In rare cases when patients have vestibular disorders in both inner ears, it could become necessary to eliminate the vestibular function in both inner ears. This could occur in bilateral Ménière's disease, one of its worst-case scenarios. Treatment is done with a medication in the same family as gentamicin (called streptomycin). Both of these medications are aminoglycoside antibiotics. If you eliminate the balance system from both inner ears, you will have completely eliminated the vestibular organ inputs. Your balance will now rely exclusively on vision and proprioception. This is clearly a deficit from which you will never fully recover. However, most patients function surprisingly well in spite of their vestibular disability. Most continue working their usual jobs provided they do not work at heights or in other precarious positions. They will be expected to have some balance problems in the dark, but most are able to walk and drive at night. They will always have some imbalance or disequilibrium with rapid head movements of any sort.

The extreme step of performing bilateral vestibular ablation is done only when vertigo attacks are so unpredictable and incapacitating that it's warranted to exchange them for some degree of chronic imbalance that is at least predictable. Streptomycin is given as a shot in an arm or buttock muscle twice daily for generally 10-14 days until the patient begins to experience quite significant disequilibrium as the endpoint.

Nondestructive Procedures

Nondestructive procedures have variable amounts of success. The general rule of thumb is that the operations with the highest success rate have more side effects. Patients desiring to minimize side effects may face lower success rates for permanent control of their vertigo.

Endolymphatic Sac Operation

Ménière's disease can be treated with an endolymphatic sac procedure. This involves opening the mastoid bone behind the ear, similarly to transmastoid labyrinthectomy, and exposing the endolymphatic sac. The sac is part of the inner ear that plays some role in regulating the pressure within the inner ear. In the past the sac was routinely opened and some type of tube or material (shunt) was placed into the sac to theoretically allow for drainage of inner ear fluids out of the inner ear in the event of excess pressure buildup. It turns out that this impression of how the operation works was far too simplistic. We now believe the operation is actually creating some type of inflammatory response that alters the physiology within the endolymphatic sac and may have a positive influence on Ménière's disease. We don't really know exactly how it works. Think of it as taking a computer that has crashed and shutting it down to reboot it. It usually works!

The recovery from this operation is generally quite fast and most patients experience no vertigo with it at all. There is no significant balance recovery period. The operation has a lower success rate, however, than the destructive procedures and most studies quote between 65-70 percent success rate in controlling, not eliminating, vertigo spells. These numbers can drop to 50-50 in studies that followed recovery three to five years after the surgery.

The operation usually will not damage the hearing but there is a risk of hearing loss with any ear operation. If the sac is opened and some type of shunt placed inside of the sac, the risk of deafness is higher than if the sac is merely *decompressed* (the overlying mastoid bone is simply removed from the sac to fully expose it). Both of these operations are equally successful in controlled studies. As a result, many surgeons have abandoned the added risks of opening the sac and inserting a shunt. It seems to add no benefit and only increases the risk of hearing loss. Some surgeons still prefer placing a shunt into the sac if they feel it improves patient's success from their own experience. If the operation were to work for a meaningful period of time and then fail, a revision operation is a reasonable consideration. If the operation were to fail early-on, then a repeat of the operation would generally not be advised.

The endolymphatic sac procedure does not burn any bridges, so it plays a controversial role in the treatment of Ménière's disease. Many surgeons will simply not perform it because it has a lower success rate than other operations and we don't really understand why it works in some cases but not others. Other surgeons favor this operation because it's not destructive. They may also site examples of patients' hearing loss fluctuations becoming stabilized after the operation whereas the destructive operations generally do not have any influence on stabilizing hearing. The promise of hearing stabilization is over-rated in endolymphatic sac surgery and it should not be used as a primary reason for recommending that operation. Statistics show that hearing stabilization rates are not as good as the vertigo stabilization rates with sac surgery.

Cochleosacculotomy

Cochleosacculotomy is a much less commonly performed procedure in which the surgeon pierces the round window of the cochlea with a pick and literally pops the swollen inner ear membranes. This is another operation in which we are uncertain exactly how it works, but the results for the relief of vertigo are reasonably good. The problem with this operation is that it causes deafness in a high rate of patients and it has a lower success rate for controlling vertigo than labyrinthectomy. The good news is that the operation generally does not cause post-operative vertigo or disequilibrium. For this reason, it's an operation favored in elderly patients with whom the doctor wishes to do a relatively short operation. It can often be achieved under local anesthesia, will not produce prolonged disequilibrium, and still has a reasonably good success rate.

Elderly patients do not compensate for post-op vertigo as quickly or as well as young people and they may experience prolonged balance recovery issues after labyrinthectomy. Active and healthy elderly patients and younger patients who are expected to recover their balance may prefer the higher success rate for vertigo relief of a transmastoid labyrinthectomy.

Intratympanic Steroid Injections

Intratympanic injection of steroids is a new procedure sometimes used for Ménière's disease. There are many different protocols for doing this and some even use elaborate slow delivery pump systems to accurately *titrate* how much medication is given to the inner ear. Studies have shown widely differing results using steroids to treat Ménière's disease and the concept is considered quite controversial. If your doctor feels there may be an inflammatory, autoimmune, or rheumatologic cause for your Ménière's disease, there may be some rationale for using this treatment in your specific condition. It is an office procedure with low risks, so some patients may have the attitude of, "Why not give it a try?"

There are various means for delivering the steroids. One involves placing a tiny absorbent wick through the eardrum and against the cochlea's round window membrane so that steroids can be delivered by patients themselves at home in a form of a steroid eardrop. This is called a *micro-wick technique*. An infusion pump to precisely deliver specific quantities of steroids through a surgically implanted catheter placed up against the round window membrane can give very accurate amounts of medication. This is a *micro-catheter technique*. Other techniques involve simply injecting the medication and allowing it to lie in the middle ear for various periods of time. Injections may be repeated every few days depending on whether you respond early on or not. All of these treatments are considered very new techniques and a lot of investigation still needs to be done to determine whether steroid injections will be helpful treatment for Ménière's disease.

Meniett Device™

The Meniett Device is a new machine that uses pressure pulsations to influence Ménière's disease. It is a sophisticated pump that resembles a common aquarium pump with a plastic tube and probe that fits air-tight into your ear. Your surgeon will need to insert a ventilating tube into your eardrum. The tube is the same type of drainage tube used to ventilate the middle ear in children with ear infection problems. Most adults can have the tube inserted as an office procedure. The device delivers specific pulsations of pressure into your ear that pass through the ventilating tube to cause some physiologic changes in the inner ear. Again, we are not sure of how the machine works, but it's thought that it may be physically shifting inner ear fluids by pressure pulses. The pulses have been researched to determine what type of pressure changes and frequencies seem to optimize the benefits.

The device is non-destructive and won't burn any bridges by trying it. It is designed for consistent usage several months at a time. You apply the pressure probe to your ear and the machine will run through a five minute cycle. You can use it one or more times daily for as many days as you feel necessary. Because it's new, we do not have any long-term studies to judge how well the device really works. A recent study indicated that about 60 percent of Ménière's patients who tried it found it of some benefit. (There is more information with a picture of the Meniett Device on page 176.)

So Many Options—How to Choose

Selecting the right procedure for you is as much a personal decision as a medical one. If your hearing is good, then you'll not want to pursue a labyrinthectomy. If your hearing is perfectly normal, you may not even wish to consider intratympanic gentamicin which in most hands has a higher risk for hearing loss than either a sac operation or vestibular nerve section. If you already have some hearing loss, intratympanic gentamicin may be a reasonable choice for you. Gentamicin injection is one of the more popular procedures because it can be done in the office and has only a moderate balance recovery process. It has a slightly lower success rate than the other destructive operations.

Clearly there is a trade-off for all of these procedures. You must weigh the issues of hearing preservation, post-treatment disequilibrium, and success rate for vertigo cure. The more destructive the procedure, the more side effects you feel afterward, but the higher your success rate. The more nondestructive a procedure, the lower the success rate but the opportunity for revision procedures is still there if the surgery fails in the long run.

Nondestructive procedures have the advantage of not burning any bridges so you may wish to try something that is nondestructive. If it doesn't work, then go on to something destructive. Other patients may feel that they've had enough of vertigo and want to go for the operation with the highest possible success rate right from the beginning and not bother with anything else. The majority of patients do prefer gentamicin for the ease of getting the treatment in the office and for the moderate balance recovery that doesn't usually force them to miss work. The procedure can be repeated if necessary and is usually not burning any significant bridges. If it doesn't work adequately, a more destructive labyrinthectomy or vestibular nerve section may be done. Generally, if a labyrinthectomy or vestibular nerve section is done after most of the balance nerve has already been eliminated by gentamicin, the balance recovery is usually quite short. The gentamicin has already done most of the damage and the destructive operation is only being done to mop up. Alternatively, endolymph sac procedure may also be done if intratympanic gentamicin fails.

There's a special type of worst-case scenario Ménière's attacks previously mentioned in this book called "drop attacks," or in the medical literature, a *Crisis of Tumarkin*. This attack is thought to be due to a disturbance of the sacculus (the neurosensory element of the vestibular organ that perceives balance in the vertical direction). Patients with drop attacks can be struck with a completely unexpected and catastrophic loss of balance that causes them to literally collapse to the ground. It's such a profound disturbance that their reflexes are often unable to protect them from a fall and they can hurt themselves, even severely. I am aware of a case in which a tractor trailer driver lost control of his rig on a highway, but fortunately no one was injured. In another case, someone fell down an ordinary flight of stairs and lapsed into a coma. One woman "dropped" while carrying a baby who miraculously fell onto her belly and was unharmed. Patients with drop attacks have been known to even drop out of a chair because they're so tremendously disoriented.

These spells are potentially life-threatening if they were to occur on stairs or operating a motor vehicle. Patients with drop attacks are forced to live with severe limitations. As it is with someone who has a seizure disorder, you should not drive, operate heavy machinery, or place yourself in any position where a sudden unexpected fall could be injurious to yourself of others. You must be extremely careful to hold on at all times on stairs. Most people don't wish to live with these types of restrictions and want to undergo an operation that will eliminate these spells as quickly and reliably as possible.

Ordinarily we want patients to undergo at least two to four months of aggressive medical therapy before we would consider them to be a medical failure and opt for some type of surgical procedure. Drop attack patients can be an exception to this. Gentamicin can be effective in the elimination of drop attacks, but the problem is that about 25 percent of treated patients might experience some recurrence of spells one, two or several years later.

In most Ménière's patients, a recurrence means they may experience some of their vertigo spells once again and they may simply request a "booster shot" or two. If the recurrence were a drop attack without any warning, the results could be devastating. One woman I treated for drop attacks did great for a couple of years and was simply walking down the street when she was struck out of the clear blue with a violent attack that caused her to collapse, smashing her face on the pavement. She looked like she'd been in a car accident, but fortunately broke no bones. It's difficult to live with this question hanging over your head after gentamicin treatment: "What if this ever happens to me?" We usually recommend labyrinthectomy or vestibular nerve section for drop attack patients early on.

If you've been treated with maximal medical therapy for your vertigo and you feel that you still don't have control of your life, you may wish to consider surgery. You certainly want to be sure that you have done everything that you can to follow conservative treatment. This would include dietary treatments if necessary, proper use of your medications, avoidance of stress and proper exercising—all in accordance with the recommendations you've been given. It is very helpful to obtain additional information from reliable sources regarding your condition and to follow those instructions as closely as possible.

If in spite of your best efforts after a few months you're still unable to control your vertigo attacks, a procedure may be reasonable for you. This is a time to involve discussion with your family, friends and coworkers. It will help you attain the best objective view on how significantly your condition is affecting you and how aggressive you should be in trying to treat it. Patients with disabling vertigo often have a great deal of frustration, fright, anxiety and even depression over their condition that is limiting their lifestyle. For this reason it's often useful to get the input of those close to you in helping you make your decision. Ultimately, it's your decision as to what you think is best.

Table 9-1 summarizes the plusses and minuses of each of the procedures in this chapter. It may give you a helpful perspective in your decision-making.

Table 9-1: Summary of Surgery for Vertigo

Labyrinthectomy

1. Surgical removal of the vestibular organ in the inner ear
2. Highest success rate for relief of vertigo
3. Intentionally deafens the ear operated
4. Prolonged balance recovery

Endolymphatic Sac Operation

1. Decompression of the endolymphatic sac that aids in regulation of inner ear fluid pressure
2. Lower success rate for relief of vertigo
3. Usually spares the hearing
4. Little or no balance recovery

Vestibular Nerve Section

1. Neurosurgical operation to selectively cut the vestibular (balance) nerve between the inner ear and the brainstem
2. High success rate for relief of vertigo
3. Usually spares the hearing
4. Prolonged balance recovery similar to labyrinthectomy

Intratympanic Gentamicin Injections

1. Office procedure to chemically deaden the balance nerve
2. Moderate success rate for relief of vertigo
3. Higher rate of hearing loss, best for patients who have pre-existing hearing loss
4. Moderate balance recovery
5. Typically involves two injections into the ear spaced one week apart. Some people require a "booster shot" one to two years after initial treatment

---

CHAPTER TEN

Vestibular Rehabilitation

Susan L. Whitney, PhD
PT, Neurological Clinical Specialist (NCS), ATC
Assistant Professor in the Departments of Physical Therapy and
Otolaryngology, University of Pittsburgh and the Centers for Rehab
Services Eye and Ear Institute, Pittsburgh, PA

Laura O. Morris, PT, NCS
Facility Director of Physical Therapy Services for the Centers for Rehab
Services, , Eye and Ear Institute, Pittsburgh, PA

Supported by NIDCD NIH DC05384 (SLW)

Dr. Whitney received her doctorate from the University of Pittsburgh and
her physical therapy education from Temple University. She is an assistant professor in physical therapy in the School of Health and
Rehabilitation Sciences and an assistant professor in the Department of
Otolaryngology at the University of Pittsburgh. She is the Program
Director of the Centers for Rehab Services Vestibular Rehabilitation
Center. Dr. Whitney has been involved for the past 12 years in an NIH-
sponsored grant related to the aging affects of the vestibular system and
has either authored or coauthored 25 papers on Medline.

Laura Morris, PT, NCS received a BS in Physical Therapy from California
State University, Long Beach. She specialized in working with neurological diagnoses prior to developing an interest in balance and vestibular disorders. In 1998, she started the Balance and Vestibular Center at Long
Beach Memorial Medical Center, a multi-disciplinary clinic working with
persons with balance and/or vestibular disorders. She has been involved
in educating physical therapy students and her peers in neurological and
vestibular subjects. In 2003, Ms. Morris received her Neurological Clinical
Specialist certification. She is involved currently in clinical research as
well as working directly with patients.

Vestibular rehabilitation is a term used for exercises commonly provided for people with balance problems, dizziness
problems or problems with balance <u>and</u> dizziness. Vestibular

rehabilitation usually is done by physical or occupational therapists who are specially trained to treat people with balance and/or dizziness problems. Typically, exercises are provided that are specifically designed to decrease dizziness and/or improve a person's balance.

When searching for a vestibular rehabilitation program for a balance disorder, you must be very careful to look for the right facility. There are many individuals who state that they can treat balance problems, but this is not necessarily true. Special training is helpful so that the therapist is better able to differentiate what your problems are and how they can be helped.

- Some important questions to ask the therapist before beginning vestibular rehabilitation might include:

- What kind of training have you had related to persons with balance disorders?

- How long have you treated people with balance disorders?

- How many patients a year do you see with balance disorders?

- Have you undergone any type of special training or extra education to better understand people with dizziness and balance problems?

These questions may be difficult for you to ask, but you can determine some of the information by asking the secretary or the scheduler about whether the practitioner has specific training in treating persons with vestibular disorders. This will be very helpful to you in determining who can provide the best care for you or someone you care about.

There are websites available that can direct you to a physical or occupational therapist who feels that they have special expertise in vestibular rehabilitation. Individuals can identify themselves on the VEDA (Vestibular Education Disorders

Association) website. Being listed on any website does not insure that the person knows a lot about people with dizziness and balance problems, but it's helpful. In addition, there is a site where physical therapists who are neurologic clinical specialists or persons who specialize in vestibular rehabilitation are listed (www.neuropt.org). Physical therapists who have special expertise in neurologic disorders often use the initials NCS (Neurological Clinical Specialist) after their name. In order to pass this special certification, they should have advanced knowledge of vestibular rehabilitation.

When searching the web for people who specialize in vestibular rehabilitation or exercises, be careful about what you're reading. It's best to look at sites that end in "org" or "edu." These sites are usually associated with organizations (org) or educational institutions (edu). Therefore, information on these sites is more likely to be accurate. One of the best sites to check is "pub med" (the National Library of Medicine- "medline" http://www.ncbi.nlm.nih.gov). The site includes summaries of current information about medical conditions and is what your doctor or therapist read. There is also an Internet resource you can visit for people who are not doctors (http://health.nih.gov). This site is written for people who have health concerns and can help you to better understand your condition. The more you know, the better prepared you are when you go to see the doctor. Often the physical or occupational therapist can help you better understand what the doctor told you.

There are many health professionals who say they can provide vestibular rehabilitation. As physical therapists we believe that physical and occupational therapists are best suited to perform most of the aspects of vestibular rehabilitation. Audiologists, at times, do the particle repositioning for benign paroxysmal positional vertigo (BPPV). It's helpful to see someone who understands the entire balance system, because areas of the body besides the ear can cause imbalance problems and it is very complex. That is why physical and occupational therapists, in our opinion, are best suited to treat people with balance and dizziness problems.

A Reason for Being Seen

There are many symptoms that can make you a good candidate for vestibular (balance) rehabilitation. It's better to have dizziness that happens when you move or change position rather than to have dizziness that is present all the time, even when you don't move. Dizziness that occurs with a change of position often can be helped with vestibular rehabilitation. Constant dizziness symptoms are more difficult to improve, but a good rehabilitation program can make you stronger, improve your balance and make you less likely to fall.

Falling to the ground is a good reason to see a rehabilitation specialist about your balance. If you're falling, especially without reason, you should see your doctor so that he/she is aware of your falling problem. Falls are seen with dizziness and balance problems, but should be checked by your doctor so that he or she can attempt to determine why you are falling.

Prescription Medicines during Vestibular Rehab

Medications to give some relief from constant dizziness symptoms may be useful during vestibular rehabilitation. There is some controversy among experts that symptom relief medication may reduce the benefits of vestibular rehabilitation because it reduces your dizziness response to the exercises. However, many patients find the exercises can be better tolerated when they take medication and they will be able to put more effort into their exercises. Most physicians now agree that it's better to take the medication to better tolerate the vestibular rehab and improve more quickly. Since some vestibular suppressants may slow your recovery, some people are advised to decrease or stop their use. This decision is up to you and your doctor. The use of medicine seems to be particularly helpful if you have dizziness and a history of migraines.

Many people don't like to take medicine. Many of the medications that are used to calm the vestibular system also make people sleepy. If you're willing to work with your doctor, this can usually be adjusted. Often what happens is that the doctor just needs to decrease the dosage slightly. Then you'll feel better. Without decreasing very significant dizziness symptoms, it's difficult for vestibular rehabilitation to work in some people especially those with constant dizziness.

Intermittent versus Constant Dizziness

People who are dizzy all the time are more difficult to treat than people who have intermittent dizziness. People who have neurological conditions often have constant dizziness that can complicate things and make it more difficult to treat. If you have fluctuating dizziness, it will be more difficult for the therapist to treat you. Regardless of the type of dizziness you have, if you work with the therapist, your balance and strength can improve.

The Vestibular Rehab Clinic Visit

Persons with dizziness and balance disorders are most commonly seen in a vestibular rehabilitation clinic. You don't have to have both of these problems in order to be seen. Everyone is somewhat different so try hard not to compare yourself to others with the same diagnosis.

You'll be asked a lot of questions about your balance and dizziness during your first visit to the clinic. You'll also be asked about what testing you had prior to coming and what the results of those tests were. Bringing your MRI reports, notes from previous doctors who have treated you for your balance or dizziness problem, and any vestibular testing results is extremely helpful to the person treating you. The more information you provide the fewer questions the therapist has to ask you. Allowing the therapist to sit down and read this information prior to beginning treatment can greatly facilitate the process.

Often at balance clinics the therapist will ask you to complete questionnaires prior to beginning testing about your balance and dizziness plus general questions about your health. You might have been through all of this before, but it's extremely helpful to fill out these questionnaires honestly. Do not have a family member fill them out for you because the information will not help the therapist if you did not complete the questionnaires. These questionnaires can often help make an accurate diagnosis. By filling out these questionnaires, the therapist can more quickly begin applying an intervention that might help you get better.

There are certain things to tell the therapist that are extremely helpful. Dizziness is a symptom that may mean different things to different people. In some instances it means lightheaded or a floating sensation. Some people complain about a "pressure type" sensation in their head, or feeling like there's swelling in the head. All of these are sometimes described as dizziness.

The sensation of vertigo is something very different and it means something different to the doctor and the therapist who are examining you. Vertigo means a true sensation of spinning. It really doesn't matter much whether the room spins or you spin. Tell the therapist that you spin. How long the spinning lasts is critical information that they need to know. The number of times you get spinning symptoms and the time of day it occurs are important. Some people actually complete a dizziness diary to help guide the therapist or physician in better treating you. This information is extremely helpful and tells us a lot about your problem. Even determining the intensity, whether it's mild, moderate or severe, helps the therapist to determine what exactly the problem is.

It is very important to use the definitions as stated above for dizziness and vertigo when you're talking to your doctor. Some people state that they're dizzy when they really are feeling wobbly or off balance. If you tell the doctor the wrong word, they will send you to the wrong specialist and you won't get the care that you need.

If you're seeing a physical or occupational therapist, they'll ask you many questions about your prior medical conditions and your prior functional level. That's really important so they know how active you were prior to developing your dizziness or balance problem.

The therapist will determine how well you can feel in your hands and your feet, the strength of your muscles, arms, legs and trunk, and also whether you have normal motion in your arms and legs.

Other aspects of the evaluation that are very important include assessing your balance. This is done in many different ways. Sometimes the therapist will have you stand on both feet, sometimes on one foot, and on different surfaces plus they will ask you to walk. Most people who have balance problems have much more difficulty walking than standing still. If you have more difficulty standing still, you need to very clearly explain this to the therapist and to your doctor. There are several conditions that specifically cause difficulty in standing still, including something called *Mal de Debarquement* and *orthostatic hypotension*. These are unusual conditions, but the doctor and the therapist need to understand your complaint.

The therapist will ask you about your ability to do different tasks and whether specific movements make you dizzy. You will also be asked about whether you've fallen as a result of your dizziness or balance problem. Sometimes people fall because of their dizziness problem. If you have the feeling of spinning when you get out of bed, you have to be very careful so that you don't fall.

Testing

Often people with balance disorders have undergone testing prior to seeing a therapist for vestibular rehabilitation. One of the tests that are usually done is caloric testing. This involves having hot and cold water placed in your ear. Caloric testing is extremely important because it's the only test that can identify which ear is damaged. Therefore, it's very important to provide the results of the testing to the therapist because the results of the caloric testing can help direct the treatment and help the therapist answer your questions about your ability to get better.

Oculomotor testing is another part of the ear testing that is usually done before starting therapy. Oculomotor testing determines how well coordinated and accurate your eye movements are in finding and following a visual target. When the therapist studies the results of the oculomotor testing, it is determined whether your eyes are working in a coordinated fashion and if you need eye exercises to try to fix your dizziness problem.

In some cases people will have a test called the rotational chair test (see Chapter 3). This test is not usually seen in a typical ear, nose, and throat doctor's office because the equipment is very expensive. You only find rotational chair testing in a specialized setting. If you had a caloric weakness in both ears, the rotational chair test is extremely helpful in allowing the therapist to determine what type of exercise is most valuable for you. With weakness in both ears, it's very important to know whether the ear still responds when the rotational chair moves at different speeds. This information is critical in providing you the best of care possible.

In some settings computerized dynamic posturography is performed (see Chapter 3). This test is done while standing and helps the therapist determine what your best treatment options are. The testing itself takes about 10-15 minutes. It's not always done because insurance companies don't universally reimburse for it. It's extremely helpful in determining how to treat you and helps the therapist determine which sensory systems are working best. The test provides a printout of information (See Figure 10-1) that allows the therapist to compare performance from one day to the next. It's often used by physical and occupational therapists as a marker of improvement.

Number of Required Treatment Sessions

After completing the evaluation, the therapist must determine the number of visits over the length of time that will be necessary to help you improve. This varies greatly across the country and by setting. In some places people with balance disorders and dizziness are seen two to three times a week for 12-14 weeks. In other settings they might be seen once a week for eight to ten weeks. And lastly, at other places they might

Table 10-1: Printout of Computerized Dynamic Posturography Results.

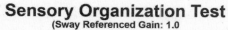

Sensory Organization Test
(Sway Referenced Gain: 1.0)

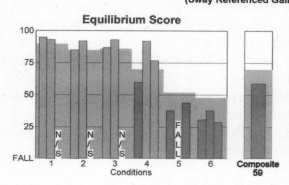

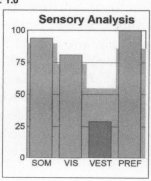

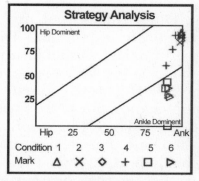

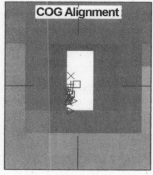

Data Range Note: User Data Range: 20–59

Post Test Comment:

be seen every two to three weeks for several months. Your frequency of visits and duration of treatment have to be determined individually based on your tests and progress with treatment. Probably even more important than the frequency of visits is having therapists skilled in vestibular rehabilitation treat you.

Home exercises are prescribed to individuals who have dizziness and balance problems. Often people who are seen more frequently have either more serious balance problems or they may be afraid of falling. It's not uncommon when people develop balance and dizziness problems that they fear they might fall. Because of this, people are sometimes seen more frequently because they may not be able to do their exercises at home alone. Some people seem to do their exercises very well at home while others need guidance. It's the decision of the therapist treating the patient as to what is the best method of care. Often people need to be seen fairly frequently to ensure that the exercises are being done correctly and that their questions are being answered.

Also, it's not uncommon for the frequency of the visits to decrease over time as treatment becomes more effective.

Home vs. Onsite Rehab Programs

With home exercises the therapist needs to be creative about what is given to you. Often things that are in your house are used as part of the exercise program. There are fancy machines that are used in balance rehabilitation that can help you improve your balance (as seen in the multiple Figures represented in Chapter 3). High tech equipment helps with improving your standing balance, but there's little data that states that it improves your balance while walking. The balance exercises given in the clinic that require movement (especially walking) are probably best for you if it's safe for you to walk. One of the things that the therapist has to decide is whether exercise is safe to do at home without falling. Often, objects are set up very carefully in the exercise instructions to ensure that you will not fall. Sometimes it's even suggested that you have a family member or friend nearby to do a particular exercise because the exercise places you at a slight risk for falling.

Sometimes the therapist has to place you at a slight risk for falling with the exercises in order for you to improve. This can produce anxiety for older adults, and that's why older persons, in particular, might need to be seen more frequently. The use of "high tech" exercise equipment is nice, but not necessarily best. A highly skilled therapist is probably much more important than the clinic having the best balance equipment in town.

The amount of time spent with the patient varies from clinic to clinic. Usually, persons with balance and dizziness problems are seen one on one or at most one on two. There are some clinics around the country that will do group exercises for people with these problems. Because you may have a problem unique to you, there needs to be some time spent one on one with you to better understand your problems and meet your needs. That's one of the questions that is really important for you to ask when looking for a therapist to treat you. If they treat multiple patients at the same time, that clinic may not be the optimal clinic for you. It takes skill to devise an exercise program for people with balance and dizziness problems because most of the time people have difficulty while walking, and the exercises in sitting or standing may not transfer into walking.

In our clinic we typically spend 45-60 minutes with each patient, each visit one on one. There are people who have excellent group programs around the country and it can work. The groups need to have similar diagnoses or some of the people may feel badly because they may not be able to do all the exercises that others can.

Developing Goals and Monitoring Progress

One of the things that you and the therapist need to do is develop goals for improvement in therapy. Typically the therapist administers walking and balance tests to determine your level of function during that session. The forms that you fill out prior to starting therapy are also vital in establishing goals. Based on the objective information that the therapist observes with your walking and balance and your completed forms, goals are established for how you're expected to function after therapy. The hope is that you'll achieve the established goals. We typically try to determine how many visits it will take to achieve these goals.

Sometimes people far exceed the initial therapy goals. It's difficult when your goals don't match the therapist's goals.

There needs to be discussion if that's the case. It helps for both the person who's dizzy or has a balance disorder and the therapist to have the same goals. Additional goals can be set after the initial ones are achieved. Just because the therapist has set what you perceive as a relatively low goal doesn't mean that you can't achieve much more.

Some of the things that enter into setting the goals include other medical problems that you might have. If you have a lot of other medical problems, it may make achieving your goals more difficult. For example, if you have migraines presently or have had a history of migraines, this will cause you to be more difficult to treat. We don't understand exactly why. We also know that if you have leg problems or leg weakness and subsequently develop a dizziness problem, it's more difficult for you to manage. Another factor that can decrease your chance of improving significantly is if you have no feeling in your feet. This sometimes occurs with *peripheral neuropathy*, which occurs most commonly with diabetes. Obviously, when you have difficulty feeling your feet it makes balancing much more difficult.

Some literature suggests that people whose vision is badly impaired will have more difficulty improving with a balance disorder. Things like glaucoma, macular degeneration, problems with contrast sensitivity and poor ability to see make it more challenging for you to get better.

Research substantiates that if you have problems in both ears, it's more difficult to improve with therapy. People who have neurological problems (like a stroke or head trauma) are also more challenging to treat. Having a disorder or injury to the brain doesn't mean that you can't get better. It just means that it may take you longer or you might not improve as much as you would like.

There are a number of things you need to tell your rehab therapist before treatment. He or she needs to know as much about your health history as possible. For example, if you have a pre-existing eye problem and then develop some weakness in the ear(s), it makes it much more difficult to treat you. If you're extremely stiff and weren't moving much before your problem started, this too will make rehab more challenging. Often people with dizziness problems start to walk stiffly and don't move much. If you were stiff to begin with (due to arthritis or other ailments) this needs to be revealed since rehabilitation could be more difficult.

Your pre-existing health conditions can cause your goals to be less than what you might have liked. In light of such challenges, you can improve, but the level of improvement will vary based on the damage that was caused to your ear(s) and/or brain.

Prognosis

Essentially, people get better from a vestibular disorder because the brain changes how it uses information from the vestibular system and other balance systems. There are three ways in which the brain helps recovery from an inner ear problem. The first two involve the brain learning to sense where you are in space differently than before. The last one involves the brain learning to keep your eyes focused while your head is moving.

If the problem is with only one inner ear, the brain learns to take altered information from the two inner ears and make sense of the altered input. The information that the brain received from one inner ear may be normal, but the information from the other inner ear may be abnormal or absent. The altered information coming from the two sides of the vestibular system is what causes dizziness. In order to recover from an inner ear disorder, the brain must get used to this new information from the two inner ears and reestablish that level as "normal." With this new level, the brain learns all over again what amount of movement is normal and stops giving you dizzy signals every time you move.

Another way that the brain helps recovery is through compensation, or substitution, of other senses. In this case, the brain uses the information that it gathers from your feet and eyes to help sense where you are in space, and compensates for the lack of information from the inner ears. Much like a blind person develops a more sensitive sense of touch, people with both inner ears affected tend to depend more upon their eyes and position of their feet or legs to tell them where they are in space.

The last way a person recovers from an inner ear disorder involves the vestibular system's role in keeping your eyes in focus while moving. The *Vestibular-Ocular Reflex* (VOR) discussed many times earlier in this book is responsible for keeping your vision clear while your head is moving. An example of this reflex at work happens when you shake your head yes or no while still keeping in focus the face of the person with whom you are speaking. Normally, the person's face doesn't jump around or come out of focus while you're nodding. If this reflex is not working as in many people with an inner ear disorder, just nodding your head can lead to blurred or jumping vision and an overall sense of imbalance.

Part of the recovery from an inner ear problem is improving the functioning of this reflex so that vision stays clear and you can focus while moving your head. The brain accomplishes this task through exercise and movement of the head, eyes and body. Some recovery of this reflex happens just by moving your head while trying to make it through the day. More rapid recovery happens by performing specific exercises that will be described later in this chapter.

The path of recovery that is utilized with any given person depends upon the specific problem. Physical or occupational therapy for vestibular problems helps to speed up the natural recovery process. In order to do so, it is essential for the therapist to know exactly what the problem is. This way, the path taken to recovery will be most beneficial and provides the best long-term results.

If you experience an inner ear disorder that only affects one ear, it's important that you focus primarily on "resetting" what the brain perceives as normal movement. If the brain never uses information from the inner ears to balance and merely substitutes with other senses (your eyes and feet), it loses out on vital information that could have been used to help you with your balance. Then, when you face a situation where the eyes and feet can't be used for keeping balance, like walking on thick carpet or sand in the dark, there's nothing left to rely on. You may think: "I'll never find myself in this situation," but you just never know.

Conversely, if someone has an inner ear disorder that affects both ears, substitution may be the most effective path to recovery. In this case, the therapist must teach the person to function as well as possible using the sensation from the feet and legs, and use the eyes to help with balance. This involves teaching balance strategies using the eyes when they are available to sense position and motion, and the feet or legs to sense position when the eyes are unavailable, like in the dark or when they're closed. The situation where people find themselves walking on the beach in twilight can be problematic. In this case, a therapist may teach patients how best to stay safe and use what they can to stay in balance and avoid situations as much as possible that will be unsafe. Use of a walking stick might avert disaster with walking on the beach at twilight.

Importance of Early Rehab Intervention

Obviously, regardless of the cause of your vestibular disorder, the sooner you begin therapy the better. Not only can a therapist make sure that you start down the right path to recovery, but therapists also can provide essential coping strategies to make recovery more tolerable. One critical strategy is that of pacing. If specific activities or chores around the house cause a tremendous amount of dizziness, then learning ways to spread those chores out over the course of a day may help keep the dizziness to a minimum and allow for more work overall to get done. Sometimes things that were very simple before have since become very difficult. The therapist can provide hints for how to manage different situations safely. A therapist can help you work through some of these issues right away and get you moving, and therefore, back to a productive life more quickly.

How Vestibular Rehab Works

Therapy for vestibular disorders takes many forms. Much of a therapist's job is to help get you moving again and manage the dizziness at the same time. Exercise and performing daily activities are the primary way of accomplishing this goal. The type of exercise utilized depends upon the unique problems that the individual demonstrates during the evaluation. Some exercises are geared toward helping with balance, some with helping the brain resolve differences in the inner ear signals, and some with improving the ability to focus. In addition, general exercise is often prescribed to improve overall physical health and well-being.

One group of exercises is used to help with specific movements that are problematic, such as turning your head or bending over to the floor. These are called "habituation" exercises. The point of these is to help the brain get used to moving and re-adjust the information from the two conflicting inner ears. The exercises, by virtue of their purpose, should cause some dizziness. By the brain continually being exposed to movement, it learns to accept those movements as part of what is "normal." The inner ears and brain become very sensitive to any head or body movement when experiencing an inner ear problem. These exercises help to desensitize the vestibular system to movement, making it better able to tolerate movement. The trick is for the exercises to cause enough dizziness for the brain to fix the problem, but not so much that it makes you miserable.

Part of the therapist's job is to figure out the right exercise dose. Examples of some exercises are turning your head, either while standing or walking, walking at various speeds, bending over, turning while walking, and lying down or sitting up quickly (see Figure 10-1). It's important to continually communicate with your therapist as to how dizzy you are with the exercises so that he or she can adjust them as needed. A good rule of thumb is that the exercises should not cause you to be dizzier than 50 out of 100 on the "dizziness rating scale" that your therapist will share with you. The dizziness should

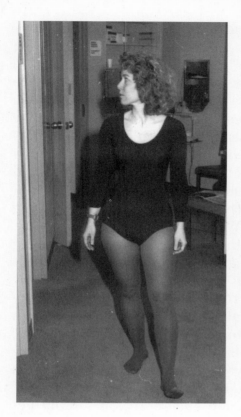 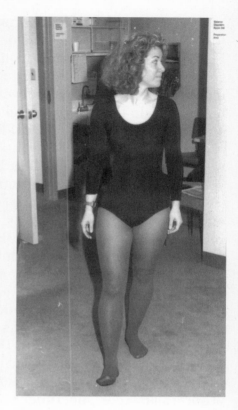

Figure 10-1: An exercise moving the head right and left while walking forward, usually given with a stop in between to look straight.

resolve within an hour or two after completing the exercises. If your symptoms are lasting longer than that or are more severe, the exercises may need to be cut back either by slowing down the movement or doing it for less time.

Balance exercises are often prescribed. Three senses are used to maintain balance: the inner ears, vision and the position sense from the feet and legs. In order to balance well, we must use information from all three systems effectively and efficiently. When one balance system is not working, our balance is affected. The goal for these exercises is to improve your ability to stand and/or move without falling. Balance exercises typically involve standing at first, then stepping or walking later as you get better.

Examples of these exercises include standing with your feet close together or with one foot in front of another (see Figure 10-2). Sometimes your therapist may have you do them with your eyes closed to encourage your feet to balance instead of relying on your eyes. Your therapist will not try to make you do balancing exercises that are too difficult, but he or she should make them challenging. If you can do the exercise easily, then it won't do much good. It's important that you minimize the use of your hands to help with your balance and you should make sure that you are safe so that you do not fall.

Physical and occupational therapy often include working on improving walking ability. When your balance isn't good, routine activities such as walking through a store or crossing a street can become so challenging that people are afraid to try. Traveling and walking on grass or sand may become impossible. These walking activities may improve just by practicing exercises in physical therapy. Some people with inner ear or balance problems have a difficult time turning to maneuver around objects in their path. This makes shopping or walking challenging in a crowded area. By working on turning activities, first in a quiet room, then in a busier area, other tasks like shopping become easier. If you simply get tired from walking for a short time or distance, your physical therapist may recommend a walking program. You may be asked to walk for a few minutes every day and then build up to 30 minutes or more. Often the walking program is started indoors if uneven sidewalks bother you or if the weather is bad, and moves outside as you are able.

Many people are surprised with how much better their ability to function gets with practice. A patient recently went through therapy for her balance that could barely walk across the room without losing her balance. She had been able to get out on her own to shop and visit friends, but had recently become so fearful of falling and so off balance that she rarely went anywhere. She was sad about not being able to interact with friends and frustrated at her declining abilities. By the end of her time in physical therapy, she was able to walk across a busy street by herself, go up and down curbs without

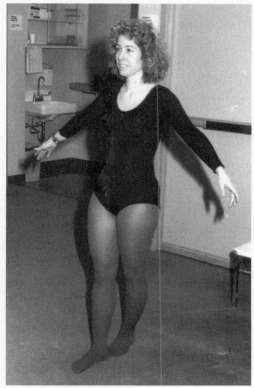

Figure 10-2: Standing with feet in front of each other.

hesitating, and manage to walk on the grass to get to her grandson's ball field. It's important to know that part of why she improved so much was that she followed her therapist's instructions and did her exercises regularly.

The last main category of exercises that may be given involves improving the coordination of your eyes and head. Some exercises involve being able to move your eyes without moving your head, or moving your head and eyes together in a coordinated fashion (see Figure 10-3). Others, called *gaze stabilization exercises*, are meant to improve your ability to keep the world still while your head is moving. These exercises involve the VOR. You may want to review some of the information in Chapter 1 that involve the reflex to refresh your memory. The VOR has some ability to improve with exercises. All of the eye-head coordination exercises usually involve

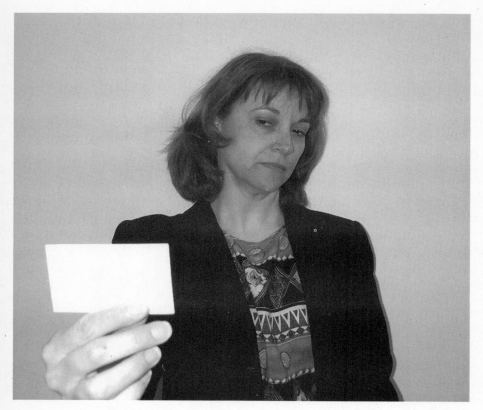

Figure 10-3: A head and eye exercise.

looking at a target, and either moving the target or moving your head. They may make you feel dizzy or nauseous, or just make your eyes tired, or both. Your therapist may ask you to first do the exercises in a quiet place so that you can concentrate and then have you try them with a busy background to make them more like real life. One patient used his wife's paisley print skirts for eye-head coordination exercises and found it worked quite well. Some patients use checkerboards or striped pieces of paper.

Your Exercise Program

The exercises that the therapist gives you to do at home will vary according to what you need to work on and how much time you can devote to exercising. It is vitally important, to the best of your ability, to do the exercises that the therapist gives you. Otherwise, it is simply not worth your time and resources to go to physical or occupational therapy. If you cannot do some of the exercises because of time constraints or their difficulty because they make you too dizzy, it's very important to communicate this to your therapist. Therapists cannot make adjustments to your program unless you tell them what you can or cannot do. Typically, the program that your therapist gives you should take no more than 20-30 minutes per day and can often be broken up into shorter time periods throughout the day. Sometimes a therapist may get carried away and give you more than you have time for in his or her enthusiasm to create your ideal program. It's your task to offer a reality check if the therapist is going overboard. What you need to know is what exercises are most important to accomplish with the time you have.

The frequency that you will be asked to do your exercises varies, often according to the goal of the exercise. You may be asked to do some exercises two to three times daily. For habituation exercises, when you're trying to get your brain to recognize normal movement as "normal," it takes reminding your brain often of what it is supposed to be doing so that the problem can be fixed. This holds true for the VOR exercises also. The eye-head coordination exercises help your brain use the VOR and other vision reflexes more effectively. Because we are trying to improve on *reflexes* (automatic connections within the brain), it's important to perform the exercises more often in order to fix them. Some therapists suggest doing gaze stabilization exercises up to five times daily. The good news is that the exercises that are to be done more frequently don't take much time. Gaze stabilization exercises usually only take two to three minutes per exercise.

Measuring Improvement

Therapists must routinely look at how you are functioning in order to know if therapy is helping. Some of this assessment happens informally, just by observing how well you walk or turn around during casual activities. Other ways to measure progress involve more formal tests and questionnaires that measure dizziness symptoms. Typically, the tests that a therapist may perform to measure your abilities on the first visit are the ones that will be repeated to measure your progress.

There is one questionnaire frequently used to measure symptoms of dizziness called the *Dizziness Handicap Inventory* (DHI) developed by Drs. Jacobson and Newman.[1] It's a series of questions about activities that may make you dizzy and how you feel when trying to function from day to day. When you complete the questionnaire, a score is tabulated and used to determine if you feel that you're getting better. There are other questionnaires that measure how confident you feel while performing various functional tasks. Your therapist may also ask you to rate the severity of your dizziness using a rating scale (like 1 to 10) in order to keep track of your symptoms.

In addition to the subjective questionnaires, many objective tests are used that measure how stable you are when walking, turning and negotiating stairs. Some also measure the speed at which you walk and perform functional tasks such as standing up and sitting down. The therapist compares your score to people without an inner ear problem in order to identify risk for falling and to help determine if you're getting better.

Prognosis

The question of your prognosis is a difficult one for a therapist to answer. Every person is different and his or her recovery from a vestibular problem is different. Some people have nearly complete recovery with no residual dizziness or balance problems, but this is less common. Most individuals have some residual dizziness, possibly only in challenging situations. People learn, through physical and occupational therapy, to manage their dizziness symptoms better in order to lead an active and productive life. A few people will have trouble with everyday functioning and may have to limit their activities in order to manage their disease. The most important way to optimize your recovery is to follow the recommendations of the medical team caring for you, including medications, exercises, activity level and pacing yourself.

There are few people who are not helped by the rehabilitation process. In order to help someone with a vestibular disorder, the first step is to assess what causes your dizziness symptoms and what makes them better. Balance and function must also be assessed. If during this process you have good balance and cannot identify any activities that increase or decrease your dizziness, then therapy is more challenging. At first there may not be a clear picture of what causes your dizziness, but over time it becomes clearer as you pay more attention to what you're doing around the time that the dizziness occurs. However, there are people for whom the dizziness occurs randomly. Those who have Ménière's disease are one example. Therapy will not have an effect on the attacks of dizziness that are common with this disease. People with Ménière's disease do find therapy helpful if they're having balance problems in between the attacks of vertigo. In these cases therapy can be beneficial.

Your therapist should be able to give you a general idea of how much better you may get after he or she has a chance to get to know you and sees how you respond to therapy in the first one or two sessions. As alluded to earlier, goals should be set for you after the first session of therapy that will reflect how much improvement your therapist hopes to achieve during your time in therapy. The important thing to realize is that there's no way to know for sure how well you will progress, and you'll usually continue to progress long after you're finished in therapy.

The amount of recovery is dependent upon several factors, some of which were discussed earlier. Those with many medical problems that complicate their health do not always recover as fully as those with originally good health. If you have a medical problem that affects other balance systems, you may have more difficulty. For example, if you have an inner ear disorder as well as diabetes mellitus that have caused nerve damage, making it difficult to feel your feet, it will be more difficult to balance than if you had the inner ear disorder alone. Those with significant visual problems such as macular degeneration or glaucoma may also have more difficulty with the recovery process.

Those individuals who have a balance or vestibular problem caused by a nerve or brain disorder have a more difficult time recovering than those whose problem is caused only by the inner ear. This category includes stroke, traumatic brain injury or any other type of brain problem that affects dizziness and/or balance. Those with a history of migraine headaches may also have more difficulty recovering from dizziness. Patients can still improve, but it may take more time and harder work. There is recent research that demonstrates that older people recover just as well as younger people, which should be good news to many.

Summary

People with balance and dizziness problems can improve with exercise. Balance, confidence and dizziness all have the potential to improve with hard work. Dizziness from inner ear problems responds to exercise when guided by a skilled rehabilitation therapist. It's not advisable to attempt to perform the exercises without supervision because you can make your condition worse. Find a good therapist you trust and work with the therapist to try and overcome your challenges.

References

1. Jacobson GP, Newman CW. The development of the dizziness handicap inventory. Arch Otolaryngol Head Neck Surg. 1990;116:424-427.

CHAPTER ELEVEN

Falls in the Elderly and Preventive Measures

Gregory F. Marchetti, PhD, PT
Assistant Professor, Department of Physical Therapy
Duquesne University, Pittsburgh, PA

Susan L. Whitney, PhD, PT
Neurological Clinical Specialist, ATC
Assistant Professor, Departments of Physical Therapy and Otolaryngology
University of Pittsburgh and the Centers for Rehab Services
Eye and Ear Institute, Pittsburgh, PA

Supported in part by NIH DC05384 (SLW)

Dr. Marchetti holds a doctorate in chronic disease epidemiology from the Graduate School of Public Health at the University of Pittsburgh. His area of expertise is the study of risk factors for falls and fall-related injuries in older adults with balance disorders. He has coauthored numerous peer-reviewed publications and national presentations in the area of falls, quality of life and psychometric properties of clinical tests of balance and functional mobility in persons with vestibular system dysfunction. He also has over 20 years experience in the rehabilitation management of persons with neurological system and postural control disorders.

Dr. Whitney received her doctorate from the University of Pittsburgh and her physical therapy education from Temple University. She is an assistant professor in physical therapy in the School of Health and Rehabilitation Sciences and an assistant professor in the Department of Otolaryngology at the University of Pittsburgh. She is the Program Director of the Centers for Rehab Services Vestibular Rehabilitation Center. Dr. Whitney has been involved for the past 12 years in an NIH-sponsored grant related to the aging affects of the vestibular system and has either authored or coauthored 25 papers on Medline.

Introduction

Falling is a very common problem in older adults and can cause catastrophic results. A fall is defined when a person is unable to stay upright and ends up laying on the ground or lower surface. While it's not uncommon to fall, the consequences can be devastating for seniors. The purpose of this chapter is to provide you with a better understanding of how frequently people fall, who is at risk, what happens to people who fall, and what can be done to prevent it. This will be presented by asking questions we felt you would want answered.

How Frequently do Falls Occur?

Each year in the United States and all other parts of the western world, about three in ten adults over the age of 65 experience a fall. While many older persons will take precautions to prevent further falls, about one to two in ten adults will fall more than once a year. Among those who fall, one out of ten will have a severe injury due to falling. The older a person gets, the greater the chance that he or she will fall. The chance of falling increases to 50 percent by the time a person reaches age 80. The chance of falling gets higher for men above age 65.

What are the Consequences of Falls to Society?

In all countries in the western world, the number of persons older than age 65 is expected to increase. This means that every year, more and more people will experience a fall. There can be grave consequences to the person as result of a fall. An increase in the number of people who will fall also will significantly impact our society and our healthcare system.

Falls are the leading cause of injury-related death in the U.S. Sixty percent of the people who die as a result of falls are older than 65 years. Falls are a source of 87 percent of the fractures sustained by older adults. The injuries that occur due to falls can result in expensive hospital and nursing home care. It is estimated that over three billion dollars is spent annually caring for people who have been injured from a fall. The U.S. government has recognized the burden that falls place on our society and healthcare system. This financial burden is expected to increase as the number of older adults increases. The U.S. government has determined that preventing fall-related deaths and injuries should be a major public health goal.

What can Cause Me to Fall?

Because so many people fall and are injured each year, much research has been done with the aim at prevention. It is known that falls and injuries are probably not totally accidental. A number of risk factors have been identified that increase your chances for a fall. Recognizing these risk factors help you to take preventative measures that may keep you from falling or becoming injured. These risk factors are summarized in Table 11-1.

Unexplained falls are serious and need to be investigated by your doctor. If you tripped over your grandchild's toy, that is not nearly as serious as if you were standing and talking to your grandchild and fell to the ground without any known cause.

Is Physical Activity Good?

Staying physically active is important to maintaining good health. A body that is in the best possible shape is less likely to get sick and will recover more quickly and completely when illness strikes. Regular physical activity either through exercise or the performance of daily chores may also help prevent falls. Physical activity can improve muscle strength, heart function, balance and endurance. These are bodily functions that have been found to affect whether or not you may fall.

An inactive person not able to get around in his or her community or leave the neighborhood is less likely to fall because there are fewer risks. While it's important to stay as active as possible, it's also important to use caution. Don't take risks by doing things that may cause you to lose your balance. It's important to participate regularly in exercises or activities that you're sure you can do safely. If you're not currently active, it's not too late to start. You may, however, need professional assistance, starting with medical advice and clearance from your doctor. It may also be important to seek the advice

Table 11-1: Problems that can make you at risk for falling.

- Alcoholism
- An inability to reach forward or to the side without fear of falling or actually falling
- An inability to go from sitting to standing without using your arms
- Being on four or more medicines (See Table 11-3 for specific medicines)
- Benign paroxysmal positional vertigo (BPPV) and other vertigo conditions
- Bilateral vestibular loss (weakness in the nerve that goes to both of your ears.)
- Decreased motion in your feet
- Decreased feeling in your feet
- Decrease in blood pressure when you move from lying down to sitting up or changing position (postural hypotension)
- Diabetes
- Environmental hazards like rugs or loose wires and cords on the floor
- Fast beating of your heart while resting (tachycardia)
- Glaucoma
- Increasing age (as you age, your risk of falling does increase)
- Macular degeneration (a problem with your eyes)
- Medications that are called benzodiazepines
- Osteoporosis (weak bones)
- Parkinson's disease
- People who are experiencing depression
- Problems with depth perception
- Problems with your nerves that go to your feet (peripheral neuropathy)
- Problems remembering things
- Stroke
- Those who have lost weight after the age of 25
- Walking very slowly
- Weakness

of a physical therapist or other practitioner who is professionally trained to design exercise programs for older adults.

How Important are Vision and Mental Abilities?

Impaired vision can be a factor that can lead to falls. Your body uses your eyes to help you stay stable and well-balanced on your feet. Good eyesight is also important to recognize objects and circumstances that may cause slips and trips. If you have a condition (cataracts or glaucoma for example) that affects your vision, see your doctor and follow the advice for treatment. If you wear glasses, try to have them checked regularly. Take extra precautions walking and performing chores in low light or dark rooms or places.

The ability to think and solve problems may also contribute to your chance of falling. Feeling anxious and having difficulty with attention span and solving routine problems may increase the chance that a person may fall. If you feel sad and hopeless about your life, feel isolated from family or friends, or if you lack desire to do things you usually like to do, see your doctor. These feelings may be signs of depression, which may increase the chance of falling.

Do Previous Falls Predict Future Falls?

If you have fallen in the past one to two years, then you're at greater risk for a fall this year. The circumstances that caused that fall may still be present. Or your body may be changing in ways that are making it difficult to stay active and have good balance. Your doctor and other healthcare professionals can help you identify these factors and decide if some treatment will be helpful in preventing future falls.

How does Dizziness Contribute to Falls?

Feelings of dizziness (spinning), lightheadedness, or feeling off balance while standing and/or walking are important factors that can lead to falls. If you feel any of these symptoms it's important to see your doctor. Feeling dizzy and off balance can have many possible causes including medications, inner ear problems, heart ailments, neurological conditions and many other problems discussed in previous chapters. It is important to identify the cause of your dizziness and work on appropriate treatment to minimize your risk of falling. You should also follow the safety advice of your physician, physical therapist or other healthcare professional to reduce your chance of falling until your dizziness improve. This may include using a walking aid such as cane or walker, and clearing your house of things that may cause you to slip or trip.

Is there a Relationship Between Bladder Control Issues and Falls?

Bladder-control problems are common in up to 50 percent of older adults. This can be caused by difficulty holding urine when the bladder is full, or not being aware that the bladder is full. These conditions are more common in women than in men. People who have trouble getting to the bathroom when their bladder is full are more likely to fall. This may be because getting to the bathroom in a hurry is hampered by problems with walking or balance. If you have these problems, you should see your doctor for possible treatment options for your bladder troubles.

Is the Presence of Other Diseases a Factor in Falls?

Many diseases or conditions have been shown to increase the chance that a person will fall. The chance for falls increases greatly if a person has two or more diseases. Some diseases directly affect the ability to stay balanced (for example, Parkinson Disease, diabetes, stroke). Other diseases such as breathing or heart disease can cause weakness or lightheadedness that can cause a fall. In addition to the effects of disease, many conditions are treated with medications that can cause drowsiness, lightheadedness and decreased balance and can lead to a fall. These symptoms have been linked with blood pressure and pain medications, and medications for anxiety or depression.

The likelihood that a person will fall increases when more medications are taken. A person who takes four or more medications has more than twice the chance of falling than someone taking fewer than three. If you're seeing more than one physician, it's important that each knows every medication that has been prescribed for you. When certain medications are taken together, symptoms of decreased balance and light-headedness can result. It's best to keep an up-to-date list of all medications you're taking with you in your wallet (both prescription and over-the-counter). Also make sure your family members have your current medication list.

Is there a Greater Risk for Falls at Home?

Objects and barriers are often present in the home that can be a cause of falls for people with balance or walking problems. Studies have shown that most falls in the home occur in the bedroom, bathroom or at the front and back door. The items or conditions involved in falls can be furniture, steps, wet or slippery floors, and floor mats or rugs. Hazards in your house (loose wires or cords on the floor, frayed rugs, etc.) can cause falls. Appendix I provides a Home Safety Checklist to determine if you have any "hazards" in your house.

Poor lighting and uneven or highly polished floor surfaces can be a problem for people with decreased balance or diminished vision. It's important to perform a home safety inspection to remove these obstacles that can cause falls (see Table 11-1 and Appendix I). If you're unable to inspect your home, there may be professionals or organizations in your community who provide this service. A good source of information may be your local agency on aging or a senior citizen's center.

What Precautions can I Take at Home?

Personal articles may also cause a fall for a person with poor balance. Loose or poor fitting clothing may get caught on furniture and cause a loss of balance. Poor fitting, badly worn or non-supportive foot-ware can increase the chance of slips and trips, especially if obstacles are present in the home. A person must also be aware of the effects of their behavior if they have symptoms such as lightheadedness or dizziness. Rising too quickly from a sitting or lying position can cause a fall and should be avoided.

What can Happen if I Fall?

An older person who falls is more likely than a younger person to get injured. It is estimated that as high as two of every ten older adults living in the community are injured from a fall every year. Falls are the fifth leading cause of death and the leading cause of injury-related death in older adults. About one in every ten falls results in a serious injury. These injuries can include damage to the brain, other internal organs and bone fractures.

Five percent of all falls result in a broken bone. Almost all (87 percent) of the bone fractures affecting older adults are due to falls. Fractures of the arms, hip and spine are the common fracture injuries from a fall. The chance of breaking a bone from a fall is greater if you have brittle bones. Everyone's bones tend to get more brittle as we get older. However, some individuals with osteoporosis (a bone disease) are more susceptible to fractures. This condition is more common among women after menopause.

All fracture injuries will cause a person to have trouble performing their normal daily activities. Of these, fracture of the hip causes the greatest disruption to a person's life. Surgery and hospitalization is generally needed to repair the broken hip. A long period of rehabilitation to regain the ability to walk and to be generally mobile will be required. Recovery of the ability to walk after a hip fracture is strongly related to how well a person was getting around before the fracture. A person who was walking safely in their home and their community without help before a hip fracture has the best chance of regaining these abilities after recovery. Some people, however, do not regain the abilities to do things as they did before the hip fracture.

What's the Risk of Loss of Independence or Decreased Quality of Life?

Falls can be an important sign that a person is becoming less mobile and is having trouble taking care of oneself. A person who has fallen has been shown to be three times more likely to require a nursing home stay than someone who has not fallen. Falls are in some way related to almost 50 percent of nursing home admissions.

Falls can cause decreased mobility either as a result of injury or as a result of fear and distress after the fall. About 25 percent of people who have fallen report they avoid their usual activities in the home for fear of falling. Falls and the resulting injuries are also a source of pain, loss of confidence and decline in the abilities to perform normal daily activities. These include restricting travel, shopping and attending worship.

What Senses Help Me to Prevent a Fall?

There are three main sensory systems that help people prevent falls. The eyes, the ears and feeling from the feet and legs are critical in maintaining balance. When any of these three systems or the brain itself are damaged or affected by other conditions, there is an increased risk of falling. The eyes, ears and feet are all connected to the brain and help us maintain our balance.

If I'm Afraid of Falling is this a Problem?

Fear of falling is a significant problem. All of us to some degree are afraid of falling, especially as we age. Sometimes this fear of falling can overwhelm us. As a result, individuals will often stop doing things they're fully capable of doing. When this occurs, they are actually increasing their risk of falling. Being active is one of the best ways to prevent a fall.

There are people who are so fearful of falling that they will not leave the house without someone with them.

When you're afraid of falling, you do less of your activities throughout the day resulting in a decreased quality of life. It also leads to increased dependence on other people. This problem of being afraid of falling can absolutely overwhelm people. When older adults' fears of falling are reduced, quality of life improves.

There are certain questionnaires given to people who help doctors and healthcare professionals determine whether the person is fearful of falling. Some of these questionnaires can identify the fear objectively and then help the doctor to make appropriate recommendations for you.

Who's at Risk of Falling?

All people fall. However, the consequences of the fall are different for older adults compared to younger people. Young people frequently fall, yet they don't face the devastating consequences of a fracture or incapacitation because of the fall. As older people age (especially into the 90s) their chance of falling significantly increases. The more active you stay, the less likely you are to fall.

Risk factors for falls are included in Table 11-1. Several of these factors will be explained.

Weakness, especially in the legs, can be a risk factor for falling. When people become weak in their legs they have difficulty walking and doing their activities of daily living. Walking is one of the best ways to ward off or prevent further osteoporosis (weak bones). Walking causes the bones to maintain or slow down the effects of osteoporosis. The muscles help the bones stay strong when they're working because they pull on the bone and that causes more bone to be produced. It is known that when people are extremely weak, their chance of falling is greater.

Those who have experienced a stroke are at a greater risk for falling as previously stated. One side of the body is often weaker than the other after a stroke. This makes people more at risk for falling depending on the severity of the stroke. There's a wide range of disability after stroke. Some people have no side effects while others can be severely incapacitated. When people have difficulty with their vision following a stroke, or have significant weakness on one side of their body, their chance of falling is much higher.

People with Parkinson's disease (progressive muscle rigidity) are at higher risk for falling. They often shuffle with their feet as they walk, having difficulty picking up their feet. Walking forward, turning and walking backward are also very difficult for people with Parkinson's disease. When walking, they are more likely to fall than persons of the same age without the disease.

Any visual problems other than wearing glasses could potentially increase the likelihood of falling. For example, macular degeneration (progressive loss of central vision) is an eye problem that makes things look darker. Walking is much more difficult without adequate light coming in through the eye to the brain. Other visual problems can also cause people to be more likely to fall, including difficulty with depth perception or glaucoma.

When people have weakness in both nerves that go to the ear, it's called bilateral vestibular loss. This has to do with the fact that one of their three main sensory systems (eyes, ears and feet) are damaged. When the ears on both sides are damaged, the eyes and the feet must try and compensate for this problem. This is somewhat overwhelming for the body to do and because of this persons with balance nerve damage in both ears are more likely to fall, especially in the dark or on uneven surfaces.

When ankles get stiff or swollen, it increases your likelihood of falling. When the ankles cannot move through the motions that they're designed to move through, individuals may fall.

If people can't feel in their feet, their chance of falling is much greater. Two common conditions that cause this are peripheral neuropathies and diabetes. Both of these are conditions that cause your feet to be numb. As a result, the eyes and ears must compensate for not getting the information about where your foot is on the ground. This can be very difficult, especially if you have visual problems or have a weakness in the nerve(s) to your ear(s).

Those who make poor judgments or have significant memory problems are at greater risk for falling. When people take multiple medications, their chance of falling is much greater. Certain types of medications are much more likely to cause a fall than others. A group of medications called benzodiazepines and sedatives have been linked to falling in older persons. Table 11-2 describes some of the medications that can place you at increased risk for falling. You should not stop taking any of these medications without consulting your doctor.

One of the easiest ways to check to see if you're at risk for falling is to try to move from sitting to standing without using your arms. Many people actually laugh when asked to do this because they're sure that they're unable to do it. It's unusual for people not to be able to get out of a standard high chair. When you have to start worrying about where you sit and whether you can get out of the couch at someone's house, you have a problem and are at increased risk for falling. The inability to get out of the chair without using your arms has been correlated to increased falls. This has to do with the fact that your legs are weak. It also can be related to fear because you may be worried about shifting far enough forward to stand up.

Walking slowly is not a good idea. Your chance of falling is actually higher than if you walk at a normal speed or slightly faster. It takes a lot more control to walk slower than it does to walk faster. If you ask a young person to walk very, very slow, you'll see that they have difficulty with their balance. This also occurs in older people. Older adults often decide to try to slow down because they think it's the best way to decrease their chance of falling, when in fact it increases their risk. Trying to get back to your normal speed of walking is a much better strategy. This has to be done carefully and with good judgment in a safe area such as a long hallway in your home.

Postural hypotension (also called *orthostatic hypotension*) is the name for a drop in blood pressure when you change positions. Such people are at higher risk for falling. If you have this problem and sense that your blood pressure is dropping or you feel faint when you change your body position, you need to talk to your doctor. There are some medications that can be prescribed that can help you control your blood pressure so that it's more stable when you change position.

When your heart beats quickly at rest (tachycardia), you're at higher risk for falling. It's important to talk to your doctor and try to see if you can get the tachycardia under control to decrease your risk of falling.

People who are fearful of reaching forward or to the side or actually fall when they reach are at higher risk for having a catastrophic fall. This has to do with many different factors, some of which include weakness in the ankles, motion problems in the ankles or the legs, or any of the problems that have previously been discussed.

Alcoholism or being a closet drinker can also increase your risk of falling because your judgment can be impaired. It's not uncommon for older adults to have an evening cocktail.

Table 11-2: Medicines that can increase your risk of falling.

- Antihistamines
- Chest pain medicine (angina)
- Medicines for anesthesia
- Medicine for anxiety
- Medicine for high blood pressure
- Medicine for pain (narcotic and non narcotic medicines)
- Medicine for psychosis
- Muscle relaxants
- Sleeping pills
- Water pills (diuretics)

However, when the evening cocktail becomes a few, that's when your chance of falling might actually increase.

As we age, the chance of falling increases. Fifty-one percent of older adults over 85 years of age have reported falling.

Those who have benign paroxysmal positional vertigo (BPPV) and other vertigo conditions are at a higher risk of falling. Vertigo causes a sudden unexpected loss of balance that could result in a fall. Unfortunately, a fall with a blow to the head could loosen up some of the inner ear crystals (*otoconia*) and create BPPV.

Those who have weak bones (osteoporosis) are more likely to experience a break if they fall. Medicines can help to prevent and possibly even add additional bone to your body. As mentioned earlier, walking and continuing to move have also been shown to help with making weak bones stronger.

If you weigh less than what you did at 25 years of age, you are at increased risk of breaking a bone if you fall. Being too thin is not good because you have lost the padding, especially over your hips that can help prevent a fracture.

Depression may also cause some people to pay less attention to their surroundings and subsequently fall.

In summary, as the number of risk factors increases, the risk of falling also increases. Very few people only have one risk factor for falling.

How can I Prevent a Fall or Fracture?

An excellent way to prevent falls is to walk. It's also one of the best ways to prevent osteoporosis. It maintains body strength and range of motion. Some people like to walk outside, while others prefer to walk on a treadmill. Both will work, but you must be careful with starting treadmill training. You'll need specific instructions on the system (perhaps with a trainer) to be sure your performance is safe. Walking on a treadmill is often not difficult, but when getting off it may result in feeling like your legs are spongy. This is why professional guidance is essential.

Ideal treadmills have devices that stop the treadmill if you fall or lose your footing. This is very important because if you were to slip and fall, the treadmill would keep going unless you have a stopping device. If you're going to purchase a treadmill, it's also a good idea to make sure it goes slowly enough for you to get started at a comfortable walking speed. These treadmills are generally more expensive, but the ones that start at zero speed and then increase in speed are really optimal for those who are just starting to become active again.

It's recommended to try and maintain your optimal body weight. Being underweight contributes to osteoporosis because your body weighs less and your bones receive less stimulation when you move and walk. Your muscle mass also protects you with padding when you fall. Excessive body weight worsens your balance and puts unhealthy loads on your bones although the extra padding can theoretically absorb some impacts from the falls.

There is some evidence that minimizing caffeine intake may also decrease your risk of fracture. This is somewhat controversial, but if you're at high risk for falling, this is certainly something that you would want to consider.

With respect to shoe wear, there's no consensus in the literature about what is the best shoe type that will prevent a fall. It has been our experience that crepe soles are difficult for older adults to walk in because they sometimes catch on the floor. Obviously, very slippery shoes should not be worn. There are some older adults who are unable to wear flat shoes because they have tightness in their calves from wearing heels all their lives. These individuals should continue to wear heeled shoes, but may work with a physical therapist to try to get their feet back to normal.

Probably the best way to try to prevent a fall is to stay physically active. This will significantly help to maintain motion in your limbs, give you a good mental outlook and keep your body strong. Table 11-3 is a good list to keep in mind.

Table 11-3: Ways to prevent falls in your house.

- Install a grab-bar or two in the bathtub or shower
- Either pick up the throw-rugs or apply tape to make sure that they stay in position
- Use good lighting in your home (less light is associated with falling)
- Make sure that all wires or cords are picked up from the floor
- Try not to stack things on the floor that could easily fall over and create a trip hazard
- Keep flashlights in rooms so you have light if there's an emergency
- Try to get a portable telephone or cell phone and have it with you, especially if you go outside and your neighbors do not live close by
- If you have a frisky pet, try to be aware of where they are so you don't fall over them
- Open-heeled slippers can be hazardous
- Use a sturdy step ladder with a handle if you have to reach up high
- Some jobs may just be too tough for you—get help to take down the curtains, cleaning the ceilings or fixing the tile on the roof
- Install good outside lighting
- Make sure that the runners on your steps are tacked down well
- Quickly clean up spills on the floor to avoid slipping
- Try to repair cracks in the sidewalk or driveway
- At the edge of a threshold (a place where the rug and tile floor meet) make sure that the edge is not in disrepair
- If it's night and you're having difficulty getting to the bathroom in time, it might be a good idea to have a portable toilet next to the bed
- Don't run to the phone. If it's important enough the person will wait for you to get there or will call again
- If you're having difficulty getting out of a chair without using your arms, you may need to see a physical therapist. Ask your doctor to send you to a knowledgeable physical therapist.

What should I do if I'm Falling?

One caution is to avoid falling to the side. If there's anyway that you can control the fall, shift forward or backward. Falls to the side are much more likely to result in a broken hip. Also, hip pads can help decrease the chance of a fracture. These pads are anywhere between ¼ to ½ inch thick. Hip pads insert into a special pair of underwear and though there's more bulk around you, it will not increase your fall risk.

If I've Fallen—Should I tell My Doctor?

You need to inform your doctor about any fall you taken. This is important because your physician may be able to help you with preventing a future fall. If you've fallen two or more times in the last six months, your chances of falling again are significantly higher. Usually the doctor or nurse in the practice can help you work through the home safety check list, and may be able to offer some suggestions about decreasing fall risk in your home.

If you've fallen, your doctor should ask you about how you fell and what medications you're taking. Your vision, walking and balance may be examined to determine whether your legs are strong. It may also be necessary to check your coordination, heart and mental acuity to be sure your nerves are working properly. All these are in the Guidelines for the Prevention of Falls in Older Persons to assist doctors in helping you prevent future falls (published by the American Geriatric Society: www.americangeriatrics.org/products/positionpapers/Falls.pdf.

What Kind of Home Modifications Have been shown to Prevent Falls?

It is controversial as to whether home modifications help. Grab-bars help decrease the risk of falling and a slip-resistant surface in the bathroom helps. Sometimes moving furniture in your home after it's been a certain way for many years may actually increase your risk of falling because you rely on that piece of furniture to help you get to the bathroom and negotiate at certain times.

There are certain slip or trip hazards that can certainly cause falls. There appears to be some evidence that relates environmental hazards to falls. Having a new cord on the floor that hasn't been there before may be a risk factor, but if it's been there for fifty years and you're very aware of it, it may not be a problem unless you develop memory issues.

It appears that bathtub benches and raised toilet seats can help people with mobility problems in the home. These make it easier for people to continue to be independent in the bathroom.

Generally, those who fall and fracture or just fall are more likely to be admitted to long-term care or a nursing home. People underreport falls because they're afraid that their family or their doctor will push them to leave their home.

Is a Cane or Walker Advisable in order to Prevent a Fall?

This is a controversial point. There are times when canes and walkers are definitely great mobility devices that will prevent falls. They need to be used correctly and must be set at the right height. Physical therapists are well-qualified to help you with this. Canes or even walkers are often used temporarily to improve your stability. Normally, people don't like to use canes or walkers because they feel there's a stigma attached to it. This certainly should be considered, but it really can improve your mobility and decrease your risk of falling. If you or your spouse starts to have memory problems, walking devices can become a hazard. People may not remember how to use them properly and can fall over the very walking aid intended to be helpful.

Am I at Risk for Falling
If I try to do More than One Thing at a Time?

There is some preliminary evidence to suggest that if you try to do multiple tasks where your attention is diverted, you may be at slightly increased risk for falling. This is presently being studied, but we know that in people who have difficulty with their memory, their attention needs to be directed toward walking and not toward walking while talking.

What Helps Prevent Falls?

By this point you no doubt already realize how important exercise is to your well-being. There is ample evidence to suggest that exercise helps decrease your risk of falling. However, we're not sure what the best type of exercise is. T'ai Chi has received a great deal of press lately because of a study that was done in 1996 by Dr. Wolf and colleagues.[1] This study suggested that T'ai Chi reduced the risk of falling by 48 percent. Strengthening and balance exercises also decrease the risk of falling. However, there is not strong evidence in the literature to suggest that one type of exercise is better than another, or does there seem to be an established preference for the exact type of exercise, length or intensity of the exercise. Nevertheless, things that can help are: doing balance and walking exercises, strengthening exercises, and movements that increase your mobility. We also believe that if you have dizziness, performing vestibular rehabilitation exercises may decrease your risk of falling.

There is evidence that if you've fallen several times, you need to be offered long-term exercise and balance training, which generally lasts over ten weeks. Also, balance training appears to be better than just strengthening exercises.

There are several common problems, potential causes and interventions that can help prevent a fall included in Table 11-4. These are directed to help you develop some rules about what you might do if you have a particular problem that increases your risk of falling.

You should note that falls in older adults can be prevented. Taking a good look at some of the risk factors that are included in Table 11-1 will help you determine your risk of falling. You must accept that not all falls are preventable. Often, people fall because they trip and would have tripped whether they were 20 or 90. A fall that occurs with no apparent reason (an unexplained fall) could occur because of some medical condition and should be investigated by your doctor.

Summary

Falls can have very serious consequences in older adults. They should be minimized as best as possible. There are some strategies that can be used to prevent falls that have been shown to be very helpful. We wish you the best of luck with trying to decrease your chance of falling, but remember that it's not all luck. You can educate yourself about prevention.

Reference

1. Wolf SL. Sattin RW. Kutner M. O'Grady M. Greenspan AI. Gregor RJ. Intense tai chi exercise training and fall occurrences in older, transitionally frail adults: a randomized, controlled trial. Journal of the American Geriatrics Society 2003;51(12):1693-701.

Table 11-4: Problems, potential cause and interventions to prevent a fall.

Problem	Potential Cause	What to do about it to decrease the chance of falling
Fear of falling	Falls or near falls; friends telling you that they have fallen	Work on doing things that you can do safely; slowly increase your activity level
Decreased strength	Not doing things; having had a bad illness that kept you from doing things	Work on walking or lifting weights that you might have in the house with the approval of your doctor
Osteoporosis (weak bones)	Decreased activity level; family history of having bone loss	Nutrition counseling; walking; bone loss medications
Lack of feeling or decreased feeling in your feet	Diabetes; peripheral neuropathy	Take your insulin and watch your diet with diabetes; maximize your other senses (eyes and ears) for balance
Can't get out of a chair without arms	Weakness in the legs; lack of motion in your feet, knees or hips	Exercise; walking program
Walking slow	Fear of falling; weakness; problems with feeling your feet; problems with vision	Work on slowly moving faster to increase your confidence; strengthening exercises, especially at for the toes, ankle and foot; see your eye doctor

Table 11-4: (*continued*) Problems, potential cause and interventions to prevent a fall.

Problem	Potential Cause	What to do about it to decrease the chance of falling
Feeling faint	Could be from a drop in blood pressure; could be from a medicine that you are taking	Contact your doctor; medication may help with the faint feeling; get out of bed slowly
Home environment may need modifications	Throw-rugs or ripped carpet may be a trip hazard; the tub or shower may be slippery	May have to pick up the throw-rugs, repair the carpet; add grab-bars in the shower or tub; add a bathmat to the floor of the bathtub or shower
Trouble seeing	Many eye problems can cause difficulty seeing including macular degeneration, glaucoma, problems with dark adaptation and contrast sensitivity	Contact your eye doctor for a through examination
Taking 4 or more prescription medicines	Multiple medicines seem to make some people groggy or not as alert, making them more at risk for falling	Talk to your doctor to see if you need to be on all of the medicines. Sometimes they can decrease the number. Check with the pharmacist to make sure that all of the medicines can safely be taken together

Appendix I: Home Safety Checklist

		Yes	No
Housekeeping			
1.	Do you clean up spills as soon as they occur?	☐	☐
2.	Do you keep floors and stairways clean and free of clutter?	☐	☐
3.	Do you put away books, magazines, sewing supplies and other objects as soon as you're through with them and never leave them on floors or stairways?	☐	☐
4.	Do you store frequently used items on shelves that are within easy reach?	☐	☐
Floors			
5.	Do you keep everyone from walking on freshly washed floors before they're dry?	☐	☐
6.	If you wax floors, do you apply 2 thin coats and buff each thoroughly or else use self-polishing, nonskid wax?	☐	☐
7.	Do all small rugs have nonskid backings?	☐	☐
8.	Have you eliminated small rugs at the tops and bottoms of stairways?	☐	☐
9.	Are all carpet edges tacked down?	☐	☐
10.	Are rugs and carpets free of curled edges, worn spots and rips?	☐	☐
11.	Have you chosen rugs and carpets with short, dense pile?	☐	☐
12.	Are rugs and carpets installed over good-quality, medium-thick pads?	☐	☐

Appendix I (*continued*): Home Safety Checklist.

		Yes	No
Bathroom			
13.	Do you use a rubber mat or non-slip decals in the tub or shower?	❏	❏
14.	Do you have a grab-bar securely anchored over the tub or on the shower wall?	❏	❏
15.	Do you have a nonskid rug on the bathroom floor?	❏	❏
16.	Do you keep soap in an easy-to-reach receptacle?	❏	❏
Traffic Lanes			
17.	Can you walk across every room in your home and from one room to another, without detouring around furniture?	❏	❏
18.	Is the traffic lane from your bedroom to the bathroom free of obstacles?	❏	❏
19.	Are telephone and appliance cords kept away from areas where people walk?	❏	❏
Lighting			
20.	Do you have light switches near every doorway?	❏	❏
21.	Do you have enough good lighting to eliminate shadowy areas?	❏	❏
22.	Do you have a lamp or light switch within easy reach from your bed?	❏	❏
23.	Do you have nightlights in your bathroom and in the hallway leading from your bedroom to the bathroom?	❏	❏

Appendix I (*continued*): Home Safety Checklist.

		Yes	No
Lighting *cont.*			
24.	Are all stairways well lit?	❑	❑
25.	Do you have light switches at both the tops and bottoms of stairways?	❑	❑
Stairways			
26.	Do securely fastened handrails extend the full length of the stairs on each side of stairways?	❑	❑
27.	Do rails stand out from the walls so you can get a good grip?	❑	❑
28.	Are rails distinctly shaped so you're alerted when you reach the end of a stairway?	❑	❑
29.	Are all stairways in good condition with no broken, sagging or sloping steps?	❑	❑
30.	Are all stairway carpeting and metal edges securely fastened and in good condition?	❑	❑
31.	Have you replaced any single-level steps with gradually rising ramps or made sure such steps are well lit?	❑	❑
Ladders and Step Stools			
32.	Do you have a sturdy stepstool that you use to reach high cupboard and closet shelves?	❑	❑
33.	Are ladders and stepstools in good condition?	❑	❑
34.	Do you always use a stepstool or ladder that's tall enough for the job?	❑	❑

Appendix I (*continued*): Home Safety Checklist.

		Yes	No
Ladders and Step Stools *cont.*			
35.	Do you always set up your ladder or step-stool on a firm, level base that's free of clutter?	❑	❑
36.	Before you climb a ladder or stepstool, do you always make sure it's fully open and that the stepladder spreaders are locked?	❑	❑
37.	When you use a ladder or stepstool, do you face the steps and keep your body between the side rails?	❑	❑
38.	Do you avoid standing on top of a step-stool or climbing beyond the second step from the top on a stepladder?	❑	❑
Outdoor Areas			
39.	Are walks and driveways in your yard and other areas free of breaks?	❑	❑
40.	Are lawns and gardens free of holes?	❑	❑
41.	Do you put away garden tools and hoses when they're not in use?	❑	❑
42.	Are outdoor areas kept free of rocks, loose boards and other tripping hazards?	❑	❑
43.	Do you keep outdoor walkways, steps and porches free of wet leaves and snow?	❑	❑
44.	Do you sprinkle icy outdoor areas with deicers as soon as possible after a snow-fall or freeze?	❑	❑
45.	Do you have mats at doorways for people to wipe their feet on?	❑	❑

Appendix I (*continued*): Home Safety Checklist.

		Yes	No
Outdoor Areas *cont.*			
46.	Do you know the safest way of walking when you can't avoid walking on a slippery surface?	❏	❏
47.	Do your shoes have soles and heels that provide good traction?	❏	❏
48.	Do you wear house slippers that fit well and don't fall off?	❏	❏
49.	Do you avoid walking in stocking feet?	❏	❏
50.	Do you wear low-heeled oxfords, loafers or good-quality sneakers when you work in your house or yard?	❏	❏
51.	Do you replace boots or galoshes when their soles or heels are worn too smooth to keep you from slipping on wet or icy surfaces?	❏	❏
Personal Precautions			
52.	Are you always alert for unexpected hazards, such as out-of-place furniture?	❏	❏
53.	If young grandchildren visit are you alert for them playing on the floor and toys left in your path?	❏	❏
54.	If you have pets are you alert for sudden movements across your path and pets getting underfoot?	❏	❏
55.	When you carry bulky packages do you make sure they don't obstruct your vision?	❏	❏
56.	Do you divide large loads into smaller loads whenever possible?	❏	❏

Appendix I (*continued*): Home Safety Checklist.

		Yes	No
Personal Precautions *cont.*			
57.	When you reach or bend do you hold onto a firm support and avoid throwing your head back or turning it too far?	❑	❑
58.	Do you always use a ladder or stepstool to reach high places and never stand on a chair?	❑	❑
59.	Do you always move deliberately and avoid rushing to answer the phone or doorbell?	❑	❑
60.	Do you take time to get your balance when you change position from lying down to sitting and from sitting to standing?	❑	❑
61.	Do you hold onto grab-bars when you change position in the tub or shower?	❑	❑
62.	Do you keep yourself in good condition with moderate exercise, good diet, adequate rest and regular medical checkups?	❑	❑
63.	If you wear glasses is your prescription up to date?	❑	❑
64.	Do you know how to reduce injury in a fall?	❑	❑
65.	If you live alone do you have daily contact with a friend or neighbor?	❑	❑

CHAPTER TWELVE

Mastering Dizziness
And Maintaining Balance

Jeffrey P. Staab, MD, MS
Assistant Professor of Psychiatry
Departments of Psychiatry and Otorhinolaryngology
–Head and Neck Surgery
The Balance Center, University of Pennsylvania School of Medicine
Philadelphia, PA

Dr. Staab is an Assistant Professor of Psychiatry in the Departments of Psychiatry and Otorhinolaryngology – Head and Neck Surgery at the University of Pennsylvania. In addition to being a board-certified psychiatrist, Dr. Staab earned a Master's degree in bioengineering based on his research in vestibular physiology. He is one of a few psychiatrists in the world who are actively involved in vestibular research. Dr. Staab's investigations have defined the interactions between vestibular disorders, anxiety, and depression as well as the psychiatric causes of dizziness. He led the first successful studies of medication treatments for dizziness and anxiety.

Is Dizziness My Destiny?

This chapter is for people with chronic dizziness, regardless of the cause. It's also for their family members, friends, lovers, coworkers and employers. No doubt, all of you have experienced the frustration that comes with chronic dizziness. Will it ever go away? What's causing it? Is it real? You hope for an answer, but sometimes find it hard to be optimistic about the future. Is dizziness your destiny? Not necessarily. Our understanding about the causes of chronic dizziness is improving rapidly and new treatments are available that are very effective for many individuals. Of course, these new treatments do not work for everyone. Some people have to find a way to cope with their dizziness over the long term. This chapter will take you through a process of understanding chronic dizziness in order to see if some of our new insights and therapies might be right for you. If you have chronic dizziness, you owe it to yourself to learn as much as you can about mastering your symptoms. Even if your dizziness cannot be cured, it doesn't have to prevent you from enjoying your life.

I Have. . .Well, I Don't Know How To Describe It —I'm Just Dizzy

People with chronic dizziness frequently find it difficult to describe their symptoms. I ask my patients a lot of questions to help them explain what they're feeling:

- Do you have vertigo?
- Lightheadedness?
- Heavy-headedness?
- Imbalance?
- Does it come and go or is it always present?
- Is it worse when you move your head, stand up or turn around?
- Do you feel better with your eyes open or closed?
- What about grocery stores, busy malls, wide-open spaces, riding in a car, or foggy days?
- Is it worse when you're tired?
- Have you ever fallen down or fainted?

The answers to these questions are not always crystal clear, but that's okay. Sensations of chronic dizziness can be confusing and vague. No need to worry about that. As strange as it seems, this very quality of vagueness can be quite helpful from a diagnostic standpoint.

As you have learned by now, dizziness and vertigo are not the same, though many people use the two words interchangeably. Keep in mind that *vertigo* is the sensation that you're spinning or the world is turning around you. It always comes in spells. It is never a constant symptom. *Dizziness* is a sensation of being off balance, off kilter, unsteady, swaying or rocking. Some people describe it as a heavy or foggy feeling in their head. Others say that they are lightheaded.

Dizziness may last for short or long periods of time. It can be a constant sensation or come and go, making some days better than others. Patients with chronic dizziness do not always have vertigo. Some have dizziness plus vertigo. Others had vertigo in the past, but now have only dizziness. Some never had vertigo at all.

Dizziness may increase with head movements and may be worse in situations where there are a lot of visual stimuli, like at busy shopping malls or when using a computer. Most patients with chronic dizziness don't fall or faint, but all feel worse when they are tired. Many people feel dizzier when they have a head cold or nasal allergies. Some can detect changes in the weather because their dizziness increases. Women may notice that their symptoms are more intense before or during their menstrual period. The important point is that chronic dizziness is hard to explain and even harder for people without it to understand. Nevertheless, its distinctive patterns can lead to specific diagnoses and effective interventions.

Occasionally, people with chronic dizziness are treated as if they're faking. Family members, employers, insurance companies or doctors may question their truthfulness. A few patients have even asked me if their own symptoms were real! If your chronic dizziness is anything like what was described above, stick to your guns and read on. If you've never experienced chronic dizziness, try shaking your head back and forth 20 times as quickly as you can or spin around quickly for a whole minute, then continue reading. This will give you only an inkling of what it's like.

Spatial Orientation

To understand chronic dizziness, we have to start with a few concepts about human spatial orientation. Humans are mobile beings. In order to be mobile, we have to know where we are in our environment, where we're going and where things are around us. We have to know whether we're standing or sitting. We have to know how fast a car is approaching us on the street so that we can cross safely.

In other words, we have to be aware of our own orientation in space as well as the locations and movements of objects around us. Each of us constructs a spatial orientation map in our brain that contains this information. We update our maps continuously with data from three sources—our senses, our vestibular system and proprioception. We receive most of our information about objects in the environment from visual cues. Hearing, smell and touch add a few more details. The vestibular system provides us with information about our head movements in all directions and also about our orientation with respect to gravity. The force of gravity is perpendicular to the earth's surface, so we use it as a benchmark for what is vertical. Proprioception is our awareness of where our body parts are relative to one another. Remember the children's song, "The head bone's connected to the neck bone, the neck bone's connected to the shoulder bone..."

Proprioception gives us precise information about the position and movement of our bodies. It's how we know our knees are bending, our head is turning or the arms are swinging at our sides. Data from our senses, the vestibular system and proprioception are analyzed in many areas of the central nervous system including the visual cortex, other areas of the sensory cortex, vestibular nuclei, cerebellum and spinal cord, as well as the neural pathways that link them together. Most of this information is processed automatically, without any conscious effort on our part. Normally, we're aware of only a small portion of these data, only what we need to negotiate our way around in the world. The brain takes care of the rest through instinctive pathways that do their job quite well outside of our conscious awareness.

Causes of Chronic Dizziness

The conditions that cause chronic dizziness lie at the crossroads of several medical specialties, including otorhinolaryngology (otolaryngology), neurology, ophthalmology, cardiology, rehabilitation medicine and psychiatry. Because of this, people with chronic dizziness may spend months or even years visiting different doctors to try to get help. It can be very frustrating when test results fail to give a clear diagnosis and treatments help just a little bit or not at all. If you're in this situation you may feel like your doctors have failed you. That's understandable. After all, you're still dizzy. The truth is that chronic dizziness can be a tough condition to sort out. Research into its causes and treatments is advancing, but there's not enough information to guide us in all cases. Sometimes it can be very difficult to find a specific cause of chronic dizziness—but not impossible.

Three general categories of illnesses cause chronic dizziness. Category #1 includes a number of chronic medical conditions. These usually are not peripheral vestibular (inner ear) problems, but other medical conditions that interfere with balance. Category #2 consists of one-time medical problems or sporadic conditions that come and go, but leave behind persistent dizziness. Category #3 includes psychiatric illnesses. Yes, a number of psychiatric disorders can cause dizziness. That's not to say that people with chronic dizziness are crazy. In fact, those who have a psychiatric cause for their dizziness may be the lucky ones. Most psychiatric causes of dizziness respond well to treatment, often better than their medical counterparts.

Category #1: Chronic Medical Illnesses

The most common chronic medical causes of dizziness are described elsewhere in this book. They include bilateral peripheral vestibular lesions, central vestibular problems and illnesses affecting proprioception or vision. Many of these do not have a cure. Strokes, head injuries, degenerative neurological conditions and peripheral nerve damage usually cannot be reversed. The goal of treatment for these illnesses is to slow down their progression or prevent relapses. On the other hand, conditions such as orthostatic hypotension (low blood pressure on standing) can be controlled well enough to minimize the dizziness that they cause.

So what do you do if a chronic medical condition is causing your dizziness? Three things. First, you make sure that your diagnosis fully explains your symptoms. Second, you work with your doctor to control your illness as much as possible. Third, you take stock of your physical and emotional functioning. Let's go over each of these steps in more detail.

(a) Be Sure the Diagnosis Fully Explains Your Symptoms

Does your diagnosis explain <u>all</u> of your symptoms? This really is your doctor's job, but you can assist in the process. Read about your illness from a reputable source. If you've been diagnosed with one of the conditions discussed elsewhere in this book, read those sections carefully. If the descriptions fit your situation, then you can be satisfied that you and your doctor are on the right track. If most of it fits, that's okay, too. Not everyone's symptoms are the same.

However, if reading about your diagnosis leaves you puzzled or if only part of its description fits, then talk to your doctor. Together, you may have to re-think your approach. Remember, chronic dizziness can be hard to sort out, so maintain a collaborative attitude with your doctor. The hours that you spend on the Internet or in the library researching your symptoms are not a substitute for years of medical education, but you may find something that prompts you and your doctor to re-evaluate your situation successfully.

(b) Work with Your Doctor

Work with your doctor to stabilize your medical condition. Specific treatments will depend on your individual circumstances. The goals are to keep your illness from getting worse and minimize the chances of a relapse. In some cases, you may recover from most or all of your symptoms. Other illnesses cannot be stopped. For these, the goal of treatment is to preserve your ability to function as long as possible. Whichever situation applies to you, stay with your treatment plan. Many people give up too early or become disillusioned when their treatment does not take their dizziness away completely.

(c) Evaluate Your Level of Functioning

Evaluate your level of functioning as objectively as possible, both physically and emotionally. This step is vitally important and often overlooked. Even if the medical problem causing your chronic dizziness cannot be cured, treatments are available to maximize your physical functioning and minimize the emotional consequences of your symptoms. Do not underestimate the importance of addressing these issues.

Physical therapy and vestibular rehabilitation may restore at least part of your lost function and reduce your imbalance. Physical therapists also can evaluate your need for special equipment (e.g., braces, canes, handrails) to increase your safety and mobility. These interventions may keep you active, increase your confidence in your balance, and decrease the frustration and social isolation that can accompany chronic dizziness.

Emotional symptoms are a natural part of any long-term illness. Chronic dizziness is no exception. Frustration, demoralization and worry are frequently part of the picture. There will be times when you cannot think of anything but your dizziness. If these emotional reactions come and go and you can honestly say that they have not taken hold of you, then keep your support systems in place—your family, friends and faith. If demoralization and anxiety have gotten the best of you, then you may need specific treatment.

Fortunately, several excellent treatments are available. They are discussed in a moment.

Category #2: Recurrent or Transient Neurotologic Conditions

Some medical conditions cause spells of dizziness that come and go. For example, Ménière's disease, vestibular migraines and benign paroxysmal positional vertigo (BPPV) cause bouts of vertigo and dizziness that typically last for days to weeks (Ménière's), hours to days (migraine), or seconds (BPPV). If you have one of these illnesses, chances are that you have good days and bad ones. You may even have weeks or months without any symptoms at all. On the other hand, you may experience day-in-day-out dizziness, chronic sensations of imbalance and persistent hypersensitivity to motion, which are punctuated by flare-ups of vertigo. This combination of acute spells of vertigo and chronic sensations of dizziness will be discussed in much more detail in just a moment. Transient neurotologic conditions such as vestibular neuronitis, minor inner ear injuries and toxic reactions to medication have a different clinical course. They cause moderate to severe vertigo, queasiness and difficulty walking, which fade over days to weeks. Most people recover completely from these conditions, but some are left with chronic dizziness, imbalance and motion sensitivity.

At this point, you may be thinking, "Wait a minute! How can episodic or temporary illnesses cause chronic and persistent symptoms?" That's a very good question. We don't know the answer for sure, but we have a couple of hypotheses. For one thing, chronic dizziness has a curious ability to change over time. The illnesses that get it started may not be the ones that keep it going. If your symptoms are different now than they were at the beginning, you may have gone through this process of change.

Your condition may have progressed from an acute to a chronic phase. Understanding this process is important for two reasons: accurate diagnosis and effective treatment. The changing nature of dizziness can fool you and your doctors. Most people want to know how their dizziness started. This is a fair question. You should know if you have a condition that requires preventative treatment. However, in most cases, the factors that sustain your dizziness are far more important for choosing an effective treatment than the ones that started it. Treatments that work perfectly well during the acute phase may not be very effective at all for chronic dizziness.

Now back to the original question, "Why do some people develop chronic symptoms from temporary or episodic illnesses?" One theory suggests that illnesses that cause vertigo disrupt the normal functioning of the vestibular system, either peripherally in the inner ear or centrally in the brain. When the illness resolves or goes into remission, it leaves behind a vestibular deficit. The brain compensates for this deficit, but not completely, producing a situation in which vestibular signals do not match other spatial orientation cues (that is, the visual and proprioceptive inputs). This sensory mismatch is thought to produce the constant sensations of dizziness, imbalance and motion sensitivity felt by many people with chronic dizziness.

This is a very attractive hypothesis and there are several lines of evidence to support it. However, not all experts agree with it. For one thing, many people with chronic dizziness have normal balance function tests, which means that if they ever had any damage to their vestibular system, their brain has compensated for it so well that it cannot be detected. It's possible that the deficits are so small that they cannot be detected with the technology of today's tests. But if that's the case, then we're left with the idea that tiny defects produce severe, even debilitating symptoms.

The second theory involves an entirely different pathological mechanism. This theory suggests that people with chronic dizziness develop a hypersensitivity to motion stimuli that lasts long after resolution of the medical problem that triggered the initial vertigo. The development of motion hypersensitivity (a process called "conditioning") is described in more detail later. Briefly, it's a process by which the brain becomes overly sensitized to even small motion stimuli, creating a high level of vigilance about visual, vestibular and proprioceptive inputs. Several research studies support this hypothesis, too. We do not know which of these theories is more important for the transition from acute to chronic dizziness. It's possible that both theories are correct and that these two mechanisms interact with one another to produce chronic and persistent dizziness. Future research will sort this out.

For now these theories have given treatment approaches that complement one other quite nicely. To get the most out of these treatments, you must understand the difference between transient episodes of vertigo and chronic sensations of dizziness. As you read the next sections, keep this distinction in mind and remember that acute treatments are for acute symptoms, chronic treatments are for chronic dizziness.

Category #3: Psychiatric Disorders

Strange, but true, more than a dozen research studies in Europe, North America and Asia have found that psychiatric disorders cause about 25 percent of all cases of chronic dizziness. That much evidence is awfully hard to ignore. Otolaryngologists, neurologists and other clinicians use the term "psychogenic dizziness" to describe these cases, but this catchall phrase is not very informative. Effective treatment requires a more precise diagnosis. Fortunately, there's plenty of research to guide us in this regard. The most common psychiatric causes of dizziness are panic disorder and related phobias. These illnesses have two parts: prominent physical symptoms and phobic behaviors.

Let's start with the physical symptoms which often occur in sudden, severe episodes called *panic attacks*. The most common symptoms of panic attacks are chest pain, rapid or pounding heartbeat, and shortness of breath. The second most common symptoms are dizziness and lightheadedness which is why panic disorder is such a common cause of chronic dizziness. However, panic attacks rarely cause vertigo. Other physical symptoms of panic include shakiness, sweating, flushing, nausea or butterflies in the stomach, and numbness or tingling in the hands, feet or lips. These physical symptoms start suddenly and build up rapidly over about five to ten minutes.

Panic attacks also have psychological symptoms such as a fear of losing control, going crazy or dying. People with dizziness usually fear that they'll fall, pass out or wreck their cars, even though these things almost never happen during a panic attack. Some people have a strange sensation of being disconnected from their bodies or their surroundings.

Panic attacks can mimic heart attacks, asthma attacks or choking spells. Often the physical symptoms are so strong that people call 911 or go to an emergency room, only to be told their heart, lungs and ears are just fine. If you've been through this scenario, you probably were not reassured about your health for very long. Panic attacks vary considerably in frequency, from a few times a year to several times a day.

Sometimes they occur in clusters and then fade away for many weeks or months, only to return for unknown reasons.

Panic attacks may occur spontaneously, seemingly out of the blue or they may be triggered by identifiable stimuli. Activities such as looking over the edge of a balcony, driving in heavy traffic or riding a crowded elevator are common triggers of panic attacks for people with dizziness. A popular myth is that panic attacks are related to high levels of stress or overwhelming life situations. Sometimes this is true, but many people with panic disorder function very well under stress and are more likely to have panic attacks when they are quiet and relaxed.

Panic attacks are hard to ignore, but they do not last very long. Usually the worst symptoms last about 15-20 minutes, following by lingering sensations that take a few hours to resolve. Worries about the next attack can persist for a long time. Panic attacks are not always severe. Some people have mild or moderate spells with only a few physical symptoms (for example, just dizziness or lightheadedness). These are called "limited symptom attacks."

Panic attacks are bad, but they're not the most devastating part of panic or phobic disorders. Two other symptoms, "anticipatory anxiety" and "phobic behaviors" are less dramatic, but often are much more disabling. Phobic behaviors include efforts to minimize future attacks and increase feelings of safety and security. Avoidance is a common strategy—avoiding people, places and activities that are associated with dizziness or other troublesome symptoms. Patients with dizziness may avoid heights, bridges, driving, movie theaters and busy malls. Needless to say, the more things you avoid and the fewer activities you do, the smaller your world becomes and the more your symptoms take a toll on your life. When avoidance becomes widespread, it is called *agoraphobia*.

The use of safety strategies is another very common phobic behavior. Safety strategies can be simple things like running your hand along the wall when you walk down a hallway or touching a piece of furniture to steady yourself when standing. Some people rely on unnecessary safety devices such as canes or walkers. Others become so insecure about their dizziness that they don't venture out of their homes alone and will not go places where they might feel trapped or unable to call for help.

People with physical causes of dizziness may legitimately need to use safety devices, at least for awhile. However, safety aids are a bad idea for people who don't have a physical need for them. Safety strategies used for psychological reasons reinforce illness behaviors and disability. They become, quite literally, crutches—mental ones. This is an important point that you must understand, especially if you use any safety strategies that go beyond your actual physical needs.

The first problem with unnecessary safety aids is that they reinforce beliefs in illness. Every time you use one, even a simple one, you send yourself a message that you're sick. How does that happen? Well, it goes like this. You use a safety strategy because you feel dizzy. It gives you a temporary feeling of security and may even let you accomplish a few things (for example, going shopping with your spouse when you cannot go alone). However, you then attribute your success to the safety strategy, not to your own abilities. You come to depend on the illusion of safety that your strategy brings and surrender the possibility that you may have the internal fortitude to overcome your symptoms. The end result is a double-whammy. You rely on a group of unnecessary safety maneuvers and you reinforce your sense of illness and disability.

The second problem with safety strategies is a physical one. People who rely on safety maneuvers rather than their own natural balance reflexes may actually increase their physical imbalance. Think about that for a minute. None of us can consciously direct our balance systems. Can you tell your muscles exactly how to get you out of a chair and walk across a room? Can you consciously direct each and every muscle movement that's needed for those tasks? Of course not! We rely on automatic motor control strategies that are stored in our brains in order to stand, walk, bend over and so on. Our motor controls are very efficient and make the best use of our body structures. Safety strategies foul them up. Instead of walking fluidly across a room, you may walk slowly, stiffly or cautiously, holding onto someone or using a cane. This takes more work than natural movements and may actually make you less steady because it interferes with your natural balance reflexes. Then, you compound this physical error by telling yourself that your safety strategy is the solution to your unsteadiness, not its cause.

I have seen patients develop physical injuries, such as back, neck and hip strains from overusing safety strategies. Their unnatural movements injured their muscles and joints. Unnecessary safety strategies also can interfere with recovery from physical vestibular illnesses. Patients may limit their natural movements to such a degree that their brains have no real opportunity to compensate for a vestibular injury. Avoidance behaviors and safety strategies seem so perfectly logical. However, they are serious symptoms that sustain and reinforce chronic dizziness. They are poor coping strategies which have to be recognized and treated for what they are.

Anticipatory anxiety is best summed up in "what if ....?" questions:

- What if I get dizzy and crash the car?
- What if I faint in public?
- What if I fall and break my hip?
- What if I can't enjoy myself because I'm so sick?

These "what if?" questions always focus on catastrophic outcomes that are possible, but very unlikely. Yet, people plan their lives around them. They anticipate bad outcomes in advance of everything they do. In fact, they can get so caught up in their worry that it takes on a life of its own. Anticipatory anxiety also reinforces avoidance behaviors. If you worry about doing something and decide to avoid it, the worry will stop, at least for awhile. If you cannot avoid whatever is on your schedule, your "what if?" questions will set your agenda for you. They will focus your attention on your symptoms, not your activity. This is another anxiety trap, another example of a seemingly logical response to dizziness (anticipation) magnifying your symptoms. I ask patients a different "what if?" question. What if none of these catastrophes happen and life passes you by while you're waiting for them? Now that would be a real tragedy.

Some people develop phobic behaviors and anticipatory anxiety without ever having a panic attack. Others have spells of dizziness and lightheadedness without the other physical symptoms. Don't split hairs about this issue. If you recognize any of the thought patterns or behaviors described in the last few paragraphs, chances are you have a significant psychological component in your illness. This may be the sole cause of your symptoms or it may coexist with medical causes. You owe it to yourself to make a full inventory of these anxiety-related thoughts and behaviors because they're quite treatable. Many patients say, "It's not all in my head, I can't be making this up!" The reality is that sometimes stress and psychological issues can actually create these symptoms and should be addressed.

Other anxiety disorders also can cause dizziness. *Generalized anxiety disorder* (GAD) is a condition of chronic worry accompanied by various nagging physical symptoms such as insomnia, low energy, muscle tension and other symptoms including dizziness that do not have a good medical explanation. Generalized anxiety disorder is the worriers' illness. We all recognize these people as serious worrywarts. If your friends or family members call you a worrywart, then your dizziness could be linked to your anxiety.

Obsessive-compulsive disorder (OCD), post-traumatic stress disorder (PTSD), and social anxiety disorder (also called social phobia) can be associated with dizziness too, but because these illnesses occasionally cause panic attacks or generalized anxiety. Depression is quite common in people with chronic dizziness, but it does not cause dizziness. Nevertheless, people who have depression with their chronic dizziness tend to be less functional than those without depression. People with clinically significant depression may not be sad sacks weeping in the corner. Depression causes bad moods—anger, irritability, restlessness, agitation or apathy—not just sadness. Sleep and appetite changes are common.

There are two types of depression. One causes increased sleep and appetite, the other insomnia and loss of appetite. Suicidal thoughts and plans are a dangerous part of depression and require immediate medical attention. Please do not underestimate the seriousness of suicidal thoughts if you or a loved one has had them. Even well-adjusted individuals can develop a great deal of despair and feel that they cannot live with a chronic medical problem like dizziness.

I'm Not Crazy! It's Not All in My Head!

No, you're not crazy! I have never seen anyone whose dizziness was caused by psychosis. Some people thought their dizziness was going to drive them crazy, but no one has lost their marbles because of dizziness.

On the other hand, your head definitely has something to do with your symptoms. After all, that's where your brain is! Furthermore, everybody has a neck. The brain talks to the body and the body talks back. Anyone who has ever felt butterflies in their stomach (anxiety) or a broken heart (sadness) knows that their body was telling the tale of their emotional state. Let's take a closer look at this issue with regard to dizziness.

Medical writings about vertigo from the 1800s contain some of the earliest descriptions of what we now call panic attacks and agoraphobia. Physicians of that time did not know much about anxiety disorders, but they engaged in a very lively debate about the origins of vertigo and its relationships to fear and other physical symptoms such as rapid heart rate and shortness of breath.

In modern times there's ample evidence of complex interactions between physical and psychiatric conditions. As described in the last section, anxiety disorders (particularly panic and phobic disorders) may cause chronic dizziness. However, the converse appears to be even more common. One of our recent investigations found that 2/3 of patients who were diagnosed with "psychogenic" dizziness actually had a medical event that triggered their dizziness. Then, they developed anticipatory anxiety, phobic behaviors, panic attacks and/or depression as a complication of their dizziness.

Being dizzy is unpleasant and chronic dizziness is hard to ignore, regardless of the cause. I have yet to find a person who is happy about being dizzy or whose life is unchanged because of dizziness. The changes may be subtle, like walking with one hand touching the wall, or they may be dramatic like giving up a job or becoming housebound. Emotional symptoms may run the gamut from minor worry and demoralization to major anxiety and depression. Regardless of how serious they are, the behavioral and emotional symptoms that accompany chronic dizziness can be treated effectively, even if the associated medical conditions cannot be cured. Before we talk about treatment, it's important to understand the current theories about how physical and psychological mechanisms may interact to sustain chronic dizziness. Our best treatments are derived from these theories and they'll make more sense after you read the next section.

Don't Eat Lunch When the Hawk Flies Over!

Think for a moment about animal shows on television. Those of you who are as old as I am probably remember Mutual of Omaha's Wild Kingdom. The younger crowd will have to think about the Discovery Channel. Animal shows often have segments that feature a poor little creature like a field mouse minding its own business while being stalked by a predator. The mouse may be eating, drinking or engaging in other mouse activities, but if it detects a predator nearby, it will stop what it's doing and react to the potential threat. It may stop, listen and sniff the air. It may freeze motionless or it may run away. The first reaction is a vigilance response. The last two are types of fight or flight behaviors. Why does a field mouse stop eating lunch when a hawk flies over? Well, it can always eat lunch later, but if it doesn't respond immediately to the threat of the hawk, it will not be around later.

These threat responses are controlled by a part of the brain called the "central nucleus of the amygdala" (CNA). The CNA and associated brain structures function as a security system. They scan the information that reaches the brain from nerves connected to our five senses and internal organs. If a possible threat is detected in the external environment or inside our bodies, the CNA initiates an instinctive behavioral response. The possible responses are the same in field mice and humans—vigilance and fight or flight.

The CNA is hard-wired to react first and think later, despite what our mothers taught us about thinking first. The CNA's warnings may be subtle or blaring, depending on the level of threat and immediacy of danger. Also, the CNA responds to potential threats, not just actual ones. Mom and the CNA agree on this point: "Better safe than sorry."

Oftentimes, we don't notice harmless stimuli. We just tune them out. To test this, stop reading for a second and listen to the noises around you that you didn't "hear" while you were concentrating on this sentence. In contrast, the CNA calls our attention to stimuli that are new, unidentified or potentially threatening. If they're benign, we notice them for just a moment (for example, just a quick glance). More significant happenings generate a vigilance response. We look, listen, feel or investigate until we're sure that there's no real danger. Serious threats produce an immediate fight or flight response with an increase in heart rate and breathing, increased muscle tension, intense concentration on the threatening stimulus, and a readiness for self-defense or quick escape. Some people freeze. These behaviors are instinctive. We cannot stop them, but we do ratchet them up or down based on our past experiences. We also can use higher thought processes to modify them. As humans, our ability to think and reason makes us less driven by pure instincts than field mice. However, we can only adjust, not eliminate, instincts and no instincts are more powerful than the threat responses.

So, what does all this have to do with chronic dizziness? Hard scientific data are just beginning to emerge on this issue, although we do have realistic theories about the relationship between the spatial orientation system, the CNA and behaviors that are part of chronic dizziness. Neural signals about spatial orientation travel to the brain's alarm system just like other sensory inputs. The CNA analyzes this information and responds accordingly. When your dizziness flares up, the CNA calls your attention to it because of two potential threats. The obvious threat is the risk of falling. Even if you've never fallen because of your dizziness, your CNA will respond to the possibility that you could ("Better safe than sorry"). However, there's a more fundamental risk, one that involves the spatial orientation system.

If you're in a situation in which your visual, vestibular or proprioceptive signals may be erroneous or mismatched, then you may not be able to update your spatial orientation maps very accurately. This would leave you quite vulnerable. Think about a field mouse with an inaccurate spatial orientation map. How long until the hawk catches it for lunch? How safe would you be in our very mobile world with a faulty orientation map in your head? This is not to say that people with chronic dizziness become completely disoriented during a dizzy spell, but it certainly is common to feel worse when confronted with multiple visual, vestibular and proprioceptive inputs.

Patients who have suffered a vestibular illness or injury have experienced their sense of orientation and movement being out of sync with reality. Obviously, the CNA takes notice. Furthermore, the experience of dizziness, no matter what triggered it, may prime the CNA to react more strongly to balance signals in the future. Think about driving and accidentally running through a stop sign. Most people will have a minor startle response which will settle down after they realize (hopefully) that they're okay. However, they'll be more consciously aware of the next few stop signs and may experience some low-level startle symptoms when they approach the next several stop signs, until they get back into their regular driving routine.

In this example, an automatic task (stopping at a stop sign) is raised to a higher level of conscious awareness (vigilance) and becomes associated with physical symptoms (minor startle) that are not usually present during the task of stopping. Then, future exposures to the same stimulus (stop signs) may reproduce the heightened awareness and physical reactions. This is called "conditioning," a process that behavioral psychologists have studied for more than 100 years, ever since the days of Pavlov and his dogs. Brain structures closely connected to the CNA seem to play a central role in conditioning, especially when potential threats are involved. Conditioning is a very efficient and effective means of learning and it serves an important role everyday with automatic behaviors. The act of stopping at a stop sign is itself a conditioned process. We do not think through every step. The visual stimulus of a stop sign (usually) triggers the behaviors needed to stop the car.

The process of conditioning has several implications for people with chronic dizziness. It may be responsible, at least in part, for the transition from acute spells of dizziness to chronic symptoms such as persistent sensations of imbalance and hypersensitivity to visual, vestibular and proprioceptive stimuli. Let's go through the steps postulated by this theory of conditioning.

Start with an acute spell of dizziness, regardless of its cause. During an acute spell, the CNA and its associated brain structures do three things:

1. They trigger any necessary self-protective responses, everything from reaching out to steady yourself to whatever degree of fight or flight response is needed;
2. They make you consciously aware of your dizziness and increase your vigilance about your balance; and
3. They record the details of your situation—who, what, when, where, why and how the dizziness occurred.

Were you reaching up to get something off of a high shelf in the kitchen, bending over to look into a bottom desk drawer, driving through a tunnel, relaxing in a chair, and so on? They also record your responses to the situation. This is the first step of the conditioning process. Your brain instinctively links dizziness, the situation in which it occurred, and your responses. It remembers these as a stimulus-response pattern. Then, the next time you're exposed to a similar stimulus (such as next time you reach up, bend over or approach a tunnel) your brain will anticipate the move and prepare for dizziness. The CNA may trigger an advanced warning, "Pay attention! Here's where/when/why/how you were dizzy before! Don't take this situation for granted," followed by increased vigilance, "Check your balance signals! Are your visual, vestibular and proprioceptive systems OK? What are they telling you?" then a safety maneuver or two, "Don't trust your balance reflexes or you'll fall/pass out/wreck! Just steady yourself for a minute until this passes!" and maybe a little avoidance behavior, "Don't do that right now. Just stay away from it."

This is a vicious circle. The more vigilant you become about your dizziness, the more likely you are to trigger a conditioned response. The more times you have a conditioned response, the more vigilant you become about your dizziness. Anticipatory responses may begin to mimic the original pattern of the dizziness itself. Then your CNA has a chance to increase your vigilance and expand your phobic behaviors, even in situations in which you could be dizzy, but are not.

Abnormal conditioning can be reversed in two ways: conditioned responses fade over time if they are not reinforced, and they also can be corrected by re-establishing a normal stimulus-response pattern like in the stop signs example previously. However, neither of these is simple where dizziness is concerned. We cannot shut down our balance system, so abnormally conditioned responses cannot fade from a lack of reinforcement. Even when we're asleep, our brains keep tabs on our bodies' positions. This is how we avoid falling out of bed at night and why we can hit the snooze button in the morning without breaking everything on the night stand.

Daytime activities are primed to reinforce motion sensitivity in patients with chronic dizziness. Take the simple act of standing. No one can stand perfectly still. We sway when we stand because we're top heavy. Our weight is concentrated on our torso which we quite literally balance on our legs. This is an active process that requires constant visual, vestibular and proprioceptive input (actually two of the three are needed) and continuous adjustment from our postural muscles. Under normal circumstances, we interpret this constant swaying as being still and ignore the automatic adjustments that our muscles make.

However, people with conditioned motion hypersensitivity seem to be consciously aware of these movements. They feel they are swaying abnormally or the ground is rocking like a boat on water. A research group in Germany[1] recently completed an experiment that illustrates this point. They showed that patients with a type of chronic dizziness called "phobic postural vertigo" were hypersensitive to a visual stimulus that gave them the illusion that they were tipping over. They unnecessarily corrected their balance much more often than normal individuals. In a somewhat different experiment, researchers in Pittsburgh[2] showed that people with chronic dizziness and anxiety were less stable on a posture platform during conflicting visual and vestibular stimuli than normal individuals. Taken together, these experiments demonstrate the vicious circle that sustains chronic dizziness.

Conditioned motion hypersensitivity prompts unnecessary corrective actions that override normal postural reflexes, further aggravating the state of imbalance, increasing vigilance and reinforcing the conditioning process. Of course, not everyone with chronic dizziness develops high levels of conditioned motion hypersensitivity and its behavioral complications, but it's a rare person indeed who has no hint of them. Conditioning is a powerful instinctive process that usually serves us quite well, but it can go overboard causing persistent symptoms.

Treatment Options

To develop an effective plan to treat chronic dizziness, you and your doctor must address two issues. First, do you have an active medical problem that is causing your dizziness or contributing to your symptoms? Chronic dizziness may be triggered by transient, recurrent or persistent medical illnesses. With the help of your doctor, determine if you have an active medical problem that is affecting your balance system. You will not improve if you are treated for inactive medical conditions.

Second, decide if your medical problem(s) explain(s) all of your symptoms. A common pitfall is to attribute chronic symptoms to a condition that cannot cause chronic problems. Take vestibular neuronitis and BPPV as examples. Vestibular neuronitis usually resolves over several weeks. If you have chronic dizziness and your most recent exams and laboratory tests are normal, then acute treatments for neuronitis will not help you, even if you had neuronitis in the past. Similarly, therapies for BPPV, which causes only brief bouts of head-movement induced vertigo, may not improve your symptoms of chronic dizziness, even if you have BPPV.

Make sure you and your doctor have a heart-to-heart discussion about these two points. Separate your acute and chronic symptoms and carefully consider whether or not your medical circumstances explain all of your symptoms. Then, make sure that you receive up-to-date treatments for your medical problems (refer to previous chapters in this book for details). Also, remember that many medical conditions that cause chronic dizziness cannot be cured, but they can be controlled. Do not stop therapies that do not bring instant relief. On the other hand, work with your doctor to objectively re-evaluate treatments that provide no benefit.

The second issue may take a bit of soul searching, plus some honest input from your family members, friends and doctor. Do you have any psychological or behavioral symptoms of chronic dizziness? In other words, do you have conditioned motion hypersensitivity, anticipatory anxiety, phobic behaviors or depression? Any of these can sustain chronic dizziness by themselves or interact with medical problems to magnify your symptoms. It may be hard to believe that any of this psychological stuff applies to you. Maybe it doesn't. But you owe it to yourself and your loved ones to be sure about that.

The psychological and behavioral aspects of chronic dizziness can be overcome quite successfully, but they rarely go away on their own if you ignore them. Your choice here is quite simple—mastery or misery, restoring balance to your life (quite literally) or allowing your dizziness to set your agenda for you. So, examine your emotional and behavioral symptoms. Minor episodes of frustration, anger, demoralization and worry are expected. You can put these in their place by recognizing them for what they are, temporary setbacks in dealing with a chronic problem. Anything more serious than that requires specific treatment.

How can you tell the difference? There are a few ways. Tally the number of days in a week that you feel frustrated, angry, demoralized or worried. If it's more than two or three days per week, then your dizziness is exacting a considerable psychological toll on you. You're spending at least half your life in a gloomy emotional state. Next, check your basic physical functions. How are your sleep, appetite, energy level, motivation, concentration and memory? Anxiety, depression and chronic physical symptoms take a toll on these functions, too.

Finally, examine your day-in and day-out behavior for any evidence of conditioned motion hypersensitivity, anticipatory anxiety, safety maneuvers and avoidance. Keep a log of your activities for a few days and ask someone you trust to help you review it for any indications of these behavioral symptoms. If you find any psychological or behavioral symptoms, three types of treatment are available to you—medication, psychotherapy and vestibular rehabilitation. The next few paragraphs will introduce you to these therapies and review our current knowledge about how best to use them. They are quite compatible with other treatments for the common medical problems that cause dizziness.

Let's start with vestibular rehabilitation which is described more extensively in Chapter 10 in this book. Vestibular rehabilitation was developed to help patients compensate for acute physical injuries to the vestibular system. Some patients with chronic dizziness have evidence on neurotologic exam or balance function tests that they have not fully compensated for past vestibular injuries. Usually the remaining deficits are minor, but may be enough to cause persistent symptoms. Other patients have normal exams and test results, but notice that specific head movements or active visual environments aggravate their symptoms. This suggests the presence of conditioned motion hypersensitivity. Another group of patients has significantly changed their posture or gait because of dizziness. Medical illnesses and safety maneuvers cause patients to change their posture and gait. All three of these problems can be treated with a carefully planned course of vestibular rehabilitation. This is best done by a physical therapist who has been trained specifically in vestibular rehabilitation techniques.

For patients with chronic dizziness, vestibular rehabilitation functions as a type of behavioral desensitization, restoring more normal levels of motion sensitivity, reducing vigilance responses and increasing normal function and confidence in automatic balance reflexes. Research studies have shown that patients can benefit from vestibular rehabilitation even if they've been dizzy for many years. However, patients with moderate to severe levels of anxiety or depression often have trouble with vestibular rehabilitation because anxiety causes them to avoid the very exercises that can help them and depression saps their motivation. In our practice, we usually treat anxiety or depression first with psychotherapy or medication, and then have our patients complete vestibular rehabilitation. A few small research studies have shown promising results using a combination of psychotherapy and vestibular rehabilitation together.

Several types of psychotherapy (talk therapy) have been developed over the last 50 years to treat anxiety and depression. One of these, cognitive therapy, also called cognitive-behavior therapy (CBT), appears to be well-suited for patients with chronic dizziness. CBT is not like the stereotypes of psychotherapy that you may have seen on television or in the movies and it's not based on Sigmund Freud's concepts that psychiatric symptoms stem from unconscious conflicts.

Rather, the basic theory of CBT is that automatic thoughts drive your emotions and behaviors. Automatic thoughts are quick messages that we give ourselves throughout the day. They influence our assessments of situations that we encounter and generate emotional and behavioral reactions based on those assessments. Let's look at an example.

Imagine yourself planning a small birthday party for your spouse. You're in a good mood, expecting him or her to be pleasantly surprised. You go to the kitchen to bake a birthday cake and find out that you do not have any eggs. You think about going to the grocery store and you automatically say to yourself, "I can't go to the store. It always makes me so dizzy that I can't function. Now, I can't make this cake. The whole party is ruined."

Almost instantaneously your mood changes. You feel frustrated, angry and sad. You reach out to steady yourself on the counter. What just happened? Your brain picked up the stimulus of the grocery store and played out your conditioned responses to it, even though the stimulus was merely anticipated. As this happened, you jumped to the conclusions that you couldn't go to the store, you won't have a cake and the party is ruined. Furthermore, your thoughts called your attention to your dizziness and you reached out automatically to steady yourself.

If we step back and examine this situation objectively, we see that the only physical stimulus was a lack of eggs. The rest of the scenario played out in your head. The grocery store, missing cake, ruined party and dizziness exist only in your thoughts. As realistic as those thoughts might be, they are still just thoughts. They can be controlled by CBT techniques.

Now imagine a different train of automatic thoughts, "Uh-oh. No eggs. Maybe I can borrow a couple from my neighbor. If not, we'll just have a party with no cake." These thoughts would produce a much different outcome. Your emotional response would be a brief period of disappointment before you turned your attention back to getting ready for the party. Also notice that there was no focus on dizziness. CBT trains you to recognize the automatic thoughts that trigger and sustain anxiety, depression, vigilance about physical symptoms and phobic behaviors. CBT also trains you to address "What if?" questions and replace them with more realistic assessments of your circumstances. It helps you identify safety maneuvers and eliminate them.

In short, CBT can treat a wide range of psychological and behavioral symptoms that accompany chronic dizziness. However, CBT is not a panacea. It's not simply a way to look for a silver lining in the problems that you face. Rather, the skills you learn in CBT can help you reframe the automatic thoughts that trigger responses conditioned to your dizziness. CBT will not make eggs magically appear in your refrigerator, but it will increase the chances that your party will go on, even if you have to make a few compromises along the way. CBT usually is administered in 12-15 weekly or twice-weekly sessions followed by occasional visits to reinforce the skills, as needed. It is not an open-ended therapy that you attend for many months or years. We have had success in using CBT for individuals and small groups of patients with chronic dizziness over the last five years. However, it has not been tested for patients with dizziness in large research studies. A few small investigations have yielded promising results.

Our knowledge about the best medication treatments for chronic dizziness is changing rapidly. For many years, patients have been prescribed the same medications for chronic dizziness as they are for acute spells of vertigo. Some of these have been presented earlier in this book, but it's worth stating again. Medications such as meclizine (Antivert™, Bonine™) and benzodiazepines (for example, clonazepam [Klonopin™], lorazepam [Ativan™], diazepam [Valium™]) work reasonably well to suppress the symptoms of acute vertigo, but do not have long-lasting benefits for chronic dizziness.

In a medication study that we conducted on 60 patients with chronic dizziness, 2/3 had taken meclizine and another 2/3 had taken a benzodiazepine (some had taken both medications) without any long-term benefit. Patients who have recurrent spells of vertigo in addition to chronic dizziness may find these medications helpful during their acute spells. Other patients require preventative medications to limit flare-ups of illnesses such as vestibular migraines or Ménière's disease. However, more effective therapies that specifically target chronic dizziness are starting to emerge from research studies.

In the late 1990s, researchers studying the interactions between anxiety disorders and chronic dizziness suggested that a group of medications known as "selective serotonin reuptake inhibitors" (SSRIs) may be useful for treating chronic dizziness associated with anxiety. Six SSRIs are available in the United States: fluoxetine (Prozac™, Sarafem™), sertraline (Zoloft™), paroxetine (Paxil™, Paxil CR™), citalopram (Celexa™), escitalopram (Lexapro™), and fluvoxamine (Luvox™). These medications are first-line treatments for many anxiety and depressive disorders. They also are used to treat migraine headaches and *dysautonomia*—two other illnesses that may cause dizziness.

We have completed two research studies investigating the benefits of SSRIs for patients who had chronic dizziness without active medical problems causing their symptoms. In the first study, 60 patients took fluoxetine, sertraline, paroxetine or citalopram. In the second study, 24 patients took sertraline. The results were very similar. Approximately 75 percent of the patients tolerated their medication well and 75-80 percent of those who took their medication for at least four to eight weeks had an excellent treatment response. The others stopped their medication because of side effects or lack of benefit.

Most patients in these studies had anxiety or depression along with their dizziness. Their psychiatric symptoms and dizziness improved together. However, a total of 25 patients in the two studies had no psychiatric illness at all. They enjoyed the same positive results from their treatment. This suggests that SSRIs may have a direct effect on chronic symptoms of dizziness, particularly the constant 24 hours-a-day symptoms that do not respond well to other treatments.

We don't know exactly how SSRIs reduce chronic dizziness, but there are two possibilities. They may reduce the hyper-responsiveness of the CNA to motion stimuli or temper the activity of nerve cells in the vestibular nuclei that process visual, vestibular and proprioceptive signals. Additional research is needed to verify these results. We have not yet tested SSRIs against placebo pills in a double-blind research study which is the gold standard for measuring the effectiveness of medications. Nevertheless, it is very reasonable to discuss SSRI treatment with your doctor so that you can weigh the pros and cons in your case. We recommend that you begin with one-half of the usual starting dose and increase it slowly. It takes about eight to twelve weeks to achieve the maximum benefits from these medications. You cannot rush the process.

What if the Dizziness Won't Stop?

Remember, "what if?" questions are your enemy! The only one worth asking is, "What if my life passes me by while I wait for my dizziness to go away?" The sad truth is that some patients have dizziness that we cannot treat. We simply do not know enough about all the causes of chronic dizziness, let alone how best to treat them. "But what if I haven't been to the right doctor? What if I haven't tried the right treatment?" The answers to these questions can be found in this book. Sit down with your doctor and go through the chapters that fit your symptoms best. If you have been through the evaluations and treatments that are described here and have come up empty, then it's time to redirect your energy to coping with chronic dizziness. That does not mean that you give up all hope for a cure, but you have to be realistic. Medical science will move forward, but research takes time. Your life will pass you by if you sit back and wait for something new to be discovered or if you try every faddish treatment that you find on the Internet. A realistic approach is to make a yearly appointment with your doctor to update him or her on your symptoms and review any new treatments that may be available.

In the meantime, I urge you to learn from patients who have gone before you about how to deal with chronic dizziness. The recommendations that follow are from patients who have coped well. They are not based on research studies, but on the real life struggles and successes of people who know exactly what you are facing. They boil down to two concepts: master your dizziness and maintain your balance.

Mastering Dizziness

You have to set an agenda for yourself. You cannot let your dizziness do it for you. Start each morning by asking yourself, "What am I going to do today?" Do not ask, "How am I feeling today?" The first question focuses your attention on your plans, regardless of your dizziness. The second one directs your attention to your dizziness, regardless of your plans. The first question puts you in charge. The second one installs dizziness as your master. There's a world of difference between these two mindsets. In the first one, you go to bed at night with a realistic plan for the next day and then wake up focused on that plan. In the second one, you go to bed every night with no plan, hoping that you'll feel okay in the morning. If you're lucky enough to feel good when you wake up, you have no plan to take advantage of it. If you feel poorly, you have nothing to do except give up on the day and stew in your symptoms. Imagine the difference between these two mindsets over the course of a week, a month or a year. Mastery creates its own momentum, one day at a time. So does misery.

Maintaining Balance

If you suffer from chronic dizziness, you simply cannot do everything you were able to do before you got sick. Far too many people measure themselves against their "old self." This is a recipe for unending frustration. Give it up. Even if you were not dizzy, how realistic would it be to go back to the way you were one, two or more years ago? You have to make the most of your life right now.

This is where the balancing act comes in. Be realistic as you set your agenda each day. Space out your tasks. Schedule breaks. Allow time for recovery after activities that provoke your dizziness. One of my patients thought she had to give up traveling, something she loved to do. Long drives and airline flights always increased her dizziness and made her very fatigued. Then she realized that she could travel quite well if she scheduled a rest day after she arrived at her destination and another one after she returned home.

Avoid the temptation to push yourself on days when you feel better. You will guarantee bad days to follow. In the long run, you'll be much more productive if you keep a consistent, moderate and predictable schedule. This may not be possible with some jobs. Try to reach an agreement with your employer about your work schedule—steady hours, limited overtime, adequate breaks. Unfortunately, some employers cannot be very flexible, but you have the right to reasonable accommodations under the Americans with Disabilities Act.

You may have to give up some of your favorite activities. A day at the amusement park? Forget the tilt-a-whirl. The "old self" may be tempted to say, "If I can't ride what I want to ride, then I'm not going at all." Where does that leave you? At home maybe alone with dizziness as your master. Finally, and most importantly, make room for the people who are closest to you. Do not become so absorbed in your own struggles with dizziness that you build up resentments toward those in your life who are not dizzy. Chronic dizziness can drive a terrible wedge between you and your loved ones. They cannot see what you have because dizziness does not create any physical scars. However, they can understand your symptoms and help you cope if you let them. The burdens you have to bear will be lighter if you bear them with someone else.

References

1. Querner V, Krafczyk S, Dieterich M, Brandt T. Phobic postural vertigo. Body sway during visually induced roll vection. Experimental Brain Research 2002; 143(3):269-75.

2. Jacob RG, Furman JM, Durrant JD, Turner SM. Surface dependence: a balance control strategy in panic disorder with agoraphobia. Psychosomatic Medicine 1997; 59(3):323-30.

Additional Readings

Staab JP. Diagnosis and treatment of psychologic symptoms and psychiatric disorders in patients with dizziness and imbalance. Otolaryngologic Clinics of North America 2000; 33(3):617-35.

Staab JP, Ruckenstein MJ. Which comes first? Psychogenic dizziness versus otogenic anxiety. Laryngoscope 2003; 113:1714-8.

Staab JP, Ruckenstein MJ, Solomon D, Shepard NT. Serotonin reuptake inhibitors for dizziness with psychiatric symptoms. Archives of Otolaryngology Head and Neck Surgery 2002; 128:554-60.

Yardley L. Overview of psychologic effects of chronic dizziness and balance disorders. Otolaryngologic Clinics of North America 2000; 33(3):603-16.

Glossary

Acoustic neuroma: a tumor arising from the vestibular nerve that courses from the inner ear to the brain that can cause disturbances of hearing and balance. These tumors are commonly referred to as 'acoustic neuromas' although the more accurate term used to describe them is *'vestibular schwannomas'*.

Afferent nerve fibers: pass sensory information from the sensory organs centrally toward the central nervous system (spinal cord and brain).

Ageotropic nystagmus: refers to nystagmus beating away from the ground when a patient is laying down on their side (lateral position).

Agoraphobia: widespread avoidance of people, places, and activities that are associated with dizziness or other troublesome symptoms.

Aminoglycoside: a class of very powerful antibiotics most commonly used intravenously for serious infections. They may have the side effect of damaging the neurosensory receptor hair cells within the inner ear (*ototoxicity*) including both the hearing organ (*cochlea*) and balance (*vestibular organ*). Some aminoglycosides have the property that they are more likely to damage the vestibular organ than the cochlea (vestibular toxic). This property may be used to treat dysfunctional vestibular organs such as with *intratympanic gentamicin* and *intramuscular streptomycin*.

Ampulla: the dilated end of each of the three semicircular canals that contains the *crista* and *cupula*, neuro-sensory elements of the *vestibular organ*.

Angular acceleration: rotational acceleration or moving faster in a circular direction.

Angular motion: rotational motion of an object such as the head.

Antiemetics : medications to suppress nausea or vomiting.

Asymmetry: the strength of the VOR eye movements produced by rotation of the head and acceleration to the right can be compared to those produced by acceleration to the left. If these are not identical, as they should be, it indicates a vestibular weakness on one side causing the asymmetry.

Atherosclerosis: hardening and narrowing of the arteries due to accumulation of plaque within arterial walls. It is a common cause for heart attacks, strokes, and peripheral vascular disease.

Audiometry (Audiogram): evaluation of hearing with tones and speech testing. Includes the common hearing test with responding to faint tones.

Auditory Brainstem evoked Response testing (ABR or BAER): diagnostic test to record brainwaves produced in response to clicks or tones presented to the ear.

Autoimmune: inflammatory process in which the body's defense mechanisms that normally reject foreign proteins, such as viruses and bacteria, mistakenly begins to attack the body's own tissues. Examples of autoimmune disease are *autoimmune inner ear disease (AIED)* that can cause hearing loss and dizziness, and rheumatoid arthritis.

Autonomic Nervous System: the portion of the nervous system that regulates internal body functions such as blood pressure, heart rate, breathing rate, control over digestive processes, and so forth.

Balance platform testing: vestibular testing using a balance platform which measures the ability for someone to stand on a computer driven moving platform. Also called *dynamic posturography*.

Benign Paroxysmal Positional Vertigo (BPPV): vertigo induced by abnormal inner ear signals generated by particular head movements and postions. It is caused by abnormal deflection of the cupula within the semicircular canal ampullae usually due to a problem with the otoliths becoming displaced. The resulting abnormal nerve impulse tricks the brain into thinking that the head and body are moving when in fact they are not. The end result is an illusion that the environment is spinning.

Benign Positional Vertigo: generally synonymous with BPPV.

Bony Labyrinth: the outermost of the two concentric compartments of the labyrinth. It contains perilymph fluid and surrounds the internal compartment called the membranous labyrinth that contains the sensorineural elements of the inner ear and is filled with *endolymph* fluid.

Brainstem: the portion of the brain at the top of the spinal cord that provides much of the unconscious functions of our brain such as regulating heartbeat, breathing rate, blood pressure, and other autonomic functions.

Canalith: calcium based crystals (*otoconia* or *otoliths*) from the *sacculus* or *utricle* that have become displaced into a semicircular canal and may cause *Benign Paroxysmal Positional Vertigo (BPPV)*.

Canalithiasis: otoconia from the utricle or saccule that have come to rest inside a semicircular canal. These calcium crystals may be freely mobile in the semicircular canal and interfere with the normal response to head movements.

Canalith repositioning procedure (CRP or Epley Maneuver): a procedure involving certain head positions to manipulate *otoconia* or *canaliths* out of a semicircular canal when they cause *Benign Paroxysmal Positional Vertigo (BPPV)*.

Central nervous system: the brain and spinal cord. The remaining part of the nervous system involving nerves that go to the rest of the body is called the peripheral nervous system.

Central vestibular disorder: refers to a vestibular disorder within the central nervous system including the vestibular nerve to the brain or the vestibular nuclei within the brain.

Cerebellum: the portion of the brain located in the back of the head that controls motor or muscle activities and coordination.

Cerebrospinal fluid (CSF): the clear watery fluid that bathes and surrounds the brain and spinal cord. It is the fluid that is sampled during a spinal tap.

Cerebrum: largest of the three portions of the brain; includes the centers responsible for higher levels of thinking, sensation, and voluntary movement.

Cervical Vertigo: vertigo caused by neck movements or positions. Vertigo is thought to be due to compromise of blood flow through the neck to the vestibular nuclei of the brain or through proprioceptive nerves coursing through the neck.

Cognitive difficulties: changes in one's mental status causing various degrees of fatigue, confusion, difficulties with memory or arithmetic, and other mental tasks.

Compensation: a recovery process in which the brain learns to adapt to using one remaining healthy vestibular organ when an inner ear disorder affects only one ear.

Computerized tomography (CT) scan: an imaging device using x-rays and computers to create high-resolution images of the interior of a patient's body. It will visualize both bones and soft tissues.

Cranial nerves: the twelve paired nerves that exit directly from the brain. All other nerves originate off of the spinal cord or from peripheral branches off of the spinal cord.

Crisis of Tumarkin (Drop attack): a vertigo attack thought to be due to a disturbance of the *sacculus* , that neurosensory element of the vestibular organ that perceives balance in the vertical direction. Patients with drop attacks can be struck with a completely unexpected and catastrophic loss of balance that causes them to literally collapse to the ground. It's such a profound disturbance that their reflexes are often unable to protect them from a fall and they can hurt themselves, even severely.

Crista: the mound of vestibular neuroepithelium (specialized sensory nerve endings) that projects into the dilated or *ampullated* end of each of the semicircular canals. It contains the vestibular hair cells that detects motion.

Cupula: gel-like covering that caps the *crista* or vestibular neuroepithelium within the *ampullated* ends of the semicircular canals. The vestibular hair cells' *stereocilia* project into the gel that sways in response to head rotation. As the head is moved in a circular motion, such as making a turn right or left or nodding the head, the fluid within the semi-circular canals moves causing movement of the gel-like covering over the hair cells.

Cupulolithiasis: otoconia that have drifted from the utricle or saccule to become lodged in the cupula, the sensory endorgan of the semicircular canal. The additional weight of these calcium crystals is thought to interfere with normal movements of the cupula that occur with head movements.

Dexamethasone: a potent steroid that may be given orally or into the middle ear (intratympanic) in the treatment of some inner ear vertigo conditions.

Dix-Hallpike ("Hallpike") maneuver: Laying down quickly to the *supine* position with the neck fully extended over the end of the bed and the head turned 45 degrees to one side.

Diuretic: a "water pill" to increase urine output and reduce the amount of fluid in the body. Commonly used for high blood pressure and Ménière's disease.

Drop attack: see Crisis of Tumarkin

Dynamic platform posturography: vestibular testing using a balance platform which measures the ability for someone to stand on a computer driven moving platform. Also called *balance platform testing*.

Dysautonomia: A chronic disorder or dysfunction of the *autonomic nervous system* that can result in low blood flow to the brain and varying degrees of lightheadedness, dizziness, true vertigo and even fainting spells.

Dysequilibrium: a sense that one's balance or equilibrium is not functioning properly. There is not have to be a hallucination of motion. Synonym: *imbalance.*

Efferent nerve fibers: pass muscle movement (motor) commands and other signals from the central nervous system out to other parts of the body.

Electrocardiogram (EKG or ECG): diagnostic measurement of heart electrical signals from electrodes placed on the chest and limbs.

Electrocochleography (EcoG): diagnostic test recording electrical signals from the cochlea. It may be abnormal in *endolymphatic hydrops* or *Ménière's disease.*

Electroencephalogram (EEG): diagnostic test recording brainwaves from electrodes placed on the scalp. It is most commonly used to detect seizures or epilepsy.

Electronystagmogram (ENG): series of tests for central and peripheral balance functioning.

Endolymph: the fluid contained within the innermost of the two concentric chambers of the labyrinth or inner ear. This inner chamber is called the membranous labyrinth and contains and bathes the nerve endings. It is completely surrounded by an outer chamber, the bony labyrinth that contains *perilymph* fluid.

These two fluids must have strict maintenance of different salt balances and their pressures must be tightly regulated for proper balance functioning. A disturbance in the sodium balances or in the pressure can lead to profound vertigo and hearing loss.

Endolymphatic hydrops: Elevated *endolymph* fluid pressure thought to be the underlying disorder in *Ménière's disease.*

Endolymphatic Sac: a membranous sac protruding from the inner ear that contains endolymph and is thought to have an important role in regulating its pressure.

Epley Maneuver: see canalith repositioning procedure.

Etiology: a medical term for the cause of an illness.

Faint: commonly used term for an unexpected loss of consciousness, sometimes sudden enough to cause a fall to the ground.

Frenzel lenses: thick lenses that blur your vision and eliminate your natural ability to suppress your nystagmus by staring at an object in the room. They also magnify your eyes so that small degrees of nystagmus may be detected.

Fukuda stepping test: a test that involves marching in place with the eyes closed. If one inner ear is much weaker than the other, subjects will typically rotate gradually toward the weaker ear.

Gain: refers to the strength of the VOR. It is calculated as the ratio of the size of the eye movement divided by the size of the head movement. Gain is typically lower than normal only if both inner ears are weak.

Generalized anxiety disorder (GAD): a condition of chronic worry accompanied by various nagging physical symptoms, such as insomnia, low energy, muscle tension, and other symptoms, including dizziness, that do not have a good medical explanation.

Gentamicin: one of the *aminoglycoside* antibiotics that may be placed into the middle ear (*intratympanic*) to take advantage of its vestibular toxicity side effects to treat *Ménière's disease*.

Geotropic nystagmus: refers to *nystagmus* beating toward the ground when a patient is laying down on their side (lateral position).

Glycerol dehydration test: a test that attempts to improve hearing in Ménière's disease. A patient ingests glycerol to dehydrate the body (and thus relieve the inner ear fluid pressure caused by the Ménière's disease). A hearing test is then administered three hours later. If the hearing test shows an improvement in hearing, the patient is likely to have Ménière's disease.

Habituation: exercises used to help with specific head movements that are problematic, such as turning the head or bending over to the floor. They help the brain adapt to the movements by allowing for re-adjustment of information from the two conflicting inner ears. The exercises, by virtue of their purpose, should cause some dizziness.

Hallpike maneuver: see Dix-Hallpike maneuver.

Head righting response: reflex that assists us in maintaining the posture of our head position as our body is moved forward, backward, left, right, up or down. It effectively helps to maintain a straight line of vision by keeping our head horizontal as our body is moved.

Heavy-headed: a person's sense that they have a weight in their head in association with not feeling entirely mentally alert or in control of their sense of well being.

Hemorrhage: bleeding

Histamine: natural occurring substances that cause dilation of blood vessels and increase blood flow into an area of the body.

They can be given as a medication to increase labyrinthine blood flow.

Holter monitor: a portable EKG (ECG) monitor that is worn for a prolonged time, typically 24 hours. When symptoms of lightheadedness are felt, the wearer pushes a button on the monitor.

Hydrops: Elevated fluid pressure or swelling in a part of the body (also see Endolymphatic Hydrops).

Hypertension: elevated ("high") blood pressure.

Hyperventilation: excessively deep breathing that can produce lightheadedness and numbness or tingling in the hands and lips. It is usually an anxiety reaction.

Hypoglycemia: low blood sugar (glucose). It can produce a feeling of lightheadedness.

Hypotension: low blood pressure, generally sufficiently low to cause symptoms such as lightheadedness and feeling faint.

Idiopathic: the cause of a condition is unknown.

Infarction: tissue death

Intramuscular: refers to treatment placed into a muscle, usually by injection.

Intratympanic: refers to inside the middle ear. It can refer to treatments such as injection performed through the eardrum to gain access into the middle ear.

Labyrinth: the inner ear including the cochlea and vestibular (balance) organs.

Labyrinthectomy: surgical removal and destruction of the vestibular organ of the inner ear. The brain no longer receives dizzy signals from the affected ear and the unaffected ear takes over the balance function for both ears (compensates). The procedure intentionally deafens the operated ear.

Labyrinthitis: inflammation within the inner ear causing acute vertigo and hearing loss. It is thought to be most commonly caused by a virus but can sometimes be due to bacterial infections or inflammatory toxins from middle ear infections.

Light-headed: a person's sense of not feeling entirely mentally alert or in control of their sense of well-being.

Macula: the sensory organ in the utricle and saccule. It contains vestibular receptor cells connected to a sheet of calcium crystals (*otoconia*) used to perceive head movements.

Magnetic Resonance Imaging (MRI): an imaging device that uses a strong magnetic field and radio waves to create high resolution pictures of the inside of a patient's body. It is best for imaging soft tissues and fluids. Hard bone is not seen on MRI.

Mal de Débarquement: means "illness when disembarking or unloading," in French. It refers to a persistent sensation of unsteadiness after being in a moving vehicle, especially boats.

Mastoid bone: a prominent bony protrusion containing a normally air-filled sinus located just behind the ear. It is connected with the air-filled middle ear.

Membranous Labyrinth: the innermost of the two concentric compartments of the labyrinth. It contains the sensorineural elements of the inner ear and is filled with *endolymph* fluid. It is surrounded by the outer bony labyrinth that is filled with *perilymph*.

Ménière's Disease: an inner ear disorder that can cause intermittent severe vertigo spells, hearing loss in the affected ear, *tinnitus*, and a sense of fullness or pressure in the ear. It is thought to be related to the elevated *endolymph* pressure or *endolymphatic hydrops*.

Menses: a woman's period. Vaginal blood flow at the end of each menstrual cycle.

Meniett device: a pulse generator air pump to deliver pulsations into the ear as a minimally invasive treatment for *Ménière's* disease.

Migraine: an inherited condition characterized by a blood vessel spasm reducing blood flow to a part of the brain that regulates (actually suppresses) the intensity of sensory input. Headaches are common but they do not always occur. Other senses may be affected causing visual disturbances, extra sensitivity to sensory input, and can cause vertigo.

Movement Coordination Test: this test measures the involuntary responses of the balance system to things that disrupt your balance. While you are standing on a balance platform support surface, the machine will suddenly move the footplate to a small degree forward or backward. The force plate measures the quickness, strength and accuracy of your response to the size of the movement that perturbed your balance.

Multiple sclerosis (MS): an autoimmune disorder that selectively destroys the myelin insulating sheaths that surround individual nerve fibers in the brain, spinal tract, and optic nerve. The damaged myelin sheaths are then replaced by scar tissue called plaques. This loss of effective insulating sheath causes the nerves to malfunction with resulting neurological deficits that may wax, wane, and progressively worsen over time.

Myofascial pain: an abnormal tightness of the neck muscles, a condition often referred to by the term, often causes referred pain or discomfort

Neurocardiogenic syncope (vaso-vagal syncope): how the autonomic nervous system misinterprets the blood flow the body needs while standing upright while sending the wrong message to the heart and blood vessels, causing the heart to slow down and the blood pressure to fall. Long periods of standing, exercise and exposure to warm temperatures typically bring on this condition. As a result of this drop in blood flow to the brain, sufferers feel lightheaded, occasionally accompanied by nausea, and feel like they're going to faint. Some may actually fall, but usually sitting or lying down will allow this sensation to pass. For some people with this condition, a feeling of tiredness or lethargy may persist for several days after such an incident.

Neurologist: A medical doctor specializing in neurological or nervous system disorders.

Neurotologist: an ear surgeon (otologist) who has taken additional training in neurology, neurosurgery, and skull base surgery to treat advanced problems involving the ear, inner ear, and the region around the ear and the temporal bone.

Nystagmus: refers to the repeated and rhythmical oscillation of the eyes. Abnormal nerve impulses from the semicircular canals most commonly cause *jerk nystagmus*, characterized by a slow phase (slow, accelerating movement in one direction) followed by a fast phase (rapid return to the original position). The direction of the nystagmus is named after the direction of the fast phase. Nystagmus can be horizontal, vertical, oblique, rotatory, or any combination thereof. *Spontaneous nystagmus* is nystagmus occurring in the absence of any motion or visual stimulation and commonly implies a vestibular disorder on one side (unilateral). *Positional nystagmus* is caused by changing the position of the head and is usually indicative of an inner ear problem.

Oculomotor control system: systems coordinating eye movements with vestibular information to maintain clear visual imaging of the world when the head moves or a person is seeing objects in motion. It includes the *VOR* and the complimentary three eye movement control systems, *optokinetic, smooth pursuit,* and *saccades.*

Optokinetic system (OPK): the strongest of the three eye movement control systems to aid the VOR to maintain clear visual imaging of the world when the head moves or a person is seeing objects in motion. The other two eye movement control systems are *smooth pursuit* and *saccades*. The optokinetic system works to keep objects in clear focus when they repeatedly move across the visual field while the head is still or in constant motion. Repeated movement of objects across the visual field produces an eye movement called *optokinetic nystagmus* as the eyes track the moving target and then jumps to lock onto the next appearing target. An example of this is watching lines of trees pass by the side of the road from a car.

Orthostatic Hypotension: low blood pressure resulting from sitting up or standing up. The low blood pressure (hypotension) can cause symptoms such as lightheadedness, feeling faint, and imbalance. This low blood pressure results from reduced blood flow to the brain that occurs when getting up and gravity takes much of the blood to lower parts of the body. The cardiovascular system usually corrects this quickly, but medical conditions and aging can slow the corrective response. Also see: *postural hypotension*, same term.

Oscillopsia: the apparent motion of objects that are known to be stationary, during head movements. It is most commonly perceived as bobbing up and down of the horizon while walking. It is especially associated with severe loss of vestibular function from both inner ears (bilateral inner ear dysfunction).

Osteoporosis: weakness of the bone due to loss of calcium. Reduced bone density causes bones to be brittle and fracture easily. It is a common problem with aging or can occur in other conditions.

Otoconia: crystals of predominately calcium carbonate packed into a layer within the *otolithic membrane* of the *sacculus* and *utricle*, the vestibular organs for perceiving motion or forces in the vertical and horizontal planes. The sacculus senses the vertical force of gravity for example. The crystals are thought to provide some weight to the membrane that exerts force on the hair cells with vertical or horizontal movement of the head. Otoconia are the "stones", "debris" or "particles" that are responsible for both cupulolithiasis and *canalithiasis* that cause *benign paroxysmal positional vertigo (BPPV)*.

Otolithic membrane: the membrane that contains the gelatinous and calcium crystal (*otoconia*) layers overlying the vestibular hair cells within the *sacculus* and *utricle*.

Otosclerosis: hereditary condition causing bone remodeling around the inner ear. If the remodeling interferes with movement of the stapes bone bringing sound vibration into the inner ear, it can cause a hearing loss. It is called a conductive hearing loss because sounds are heard better conducted through bony parts of the head than through the ear itself.

Otologist: an ear surgeon. An *otolaryngologist* (ear, nose, and throat surgeon) who has specialized in medical and surgical treatment of ear problems.

Oto-neurologist: a neurologist who has sub-specialized in vertigo and balance disorders.

Otosclerosis: an abnormality of excessive bone growth that may cause the footplate of the stapes to become fixed to cause a *conductive* (mechanical) hearing loss. It may also affect the inner ear causing sensorineural (nerve damage) hearing loss or vertigo and dysequilibrium.

Otoscope: the handheld instrument doctors use to look into the ear.

Ototoxicity (ototoxic): certain medications have a toxic side effect on the inner ear and may cause nerve damage to the hearing, balance function or both. Medications with these toxic side effects affecting the ear are called ototoxic.

Oval window: The oval-shaped window into the cochlea that is sealed off by the stapes (stirrup) bone, which drives sound from the middle ear into the inner ear.

Panic attacks: acute uncontrollable anxiety episode with symptoms of chest pain, rapid or pounding heartbeat, shortness of breath, dizziness and lightheadedness.

Particle repositioning maneuver (PRM): a modification of the *canalith repositioning procedure* using a simplified and better tolerated three-position maneuver that generally eliminates the routine use of sedation and skull vibration.

Perilymph: the fluid contained within the outer most of the two concentric chambers of the labyrinth or inner ear. This outer chamber, the bony labyrinth, contains perilymph and completely surrounds the membranous labyrinth that contains endolymph. These two fluids must have strict maintenance of different sodium balances and their pressures must be tightly regulated for proper balance functioning. A disturbance in the sodium balances or in the pressure can lead to profound vertigo and hearing loss.

Perilymphatic fistula: perilymph fluid escaping from the inner ear and into the middle ear through a defect in the bone that normally separates the inner and middle ear. The most common sites of perilymph fluid leak are through the *oval window* or *round window* of the *cochlea.*

Peripheral Neuropathy: a decreased sensation in the arms or legs. Most commonly it occurs in the legs with a decreased sense of touch and sense of position (proprioception). It is a common complication of diabetes. Your balance system depends on the inner ear and brain balance centers, vision, and proprioception from the legs. Peripheral neuropathy contributes significantly to balance disorders.

Peripheral vestibular disorder: refers to a vestibular disorder involving the inner ear.

Phase: head movements should stimulate the VOR to produce closely matching eye movements. A vestibular disorder may disrupt the timing and bring the eye movements out of phase with the head movements and create a measurable time lag, especially with slow movements.

Phonophobia: sound is perceived as being too loud.

Photophobia: light is perceived as being too bright.

Positional vertigo: vertigo induced by head movements or certain head positions. Sometimes used synonymously with *Benign Positional Vertigo* or *Benign Paroxysmal Positional Vertigo (BPPV)* caused specifically by displaced otoliths inducing vertigo.

Posterior semicircular canal occlusion procedure: an operation to plug the posterior canal as treatment for *Benign Paroxysmal Positional Vertigo (BPPV)* that has failed conservative treatment with *particle repositioning maneuvers.*

Postural hypotension: abnormal lowering of blood pressure when raising up to a sitting or standing position. There is normally a brief drop in blood pressure when getting up quickly but it should be quickly corrected. If not, lightheadedness and feeling faint may occur.

Presbycusis: gradual loss of hearing with aging, especially in the higher frequencies.

Proprioception: sensory information from the soles of our feet and our joints (especially the ankle, knee, hip and neck) to relate to the brain the position of body and limbs in space.

Rotational chair testing: vestibular testing using a gently turning computer driven chair to mildly stimulate the balance.

Round window: a small opening into the cochlea that faces the middle ear and is covered by a thin *round window membrane.* The membrane serves to dampen out sound waves after they have passed through the cochlea after having been processed and heard.

Saccades: rapid eye movement to quickly locate and accurately lock the vision onto a target.

Saccadic system: one of the three eye movement control systems to aid the VOR to maintain clear visual imaging of the world when the head moves or a person is seeing objects in motion. The other two eye movement control systems are *optokinetic* and *smooth pursuit.* The primary function of the saccadic movements is to rapidly move the eye and position your focus on a target of interest, especially when it is moving quickly and in an unpredicted direction. This is the system that takes over for the smooth pursuit system when it can no longer keep up with the target being followed.

Saccule (Sacculus): One of the five neurosensory elements within the *vestibular organ* that senses linear motion in an upward and downward direction. The 3 *semicircular canals, utricle,* and *saccule,* comprise the five neurosensory elements within the *vestibular organ* or balance organ within the inner ear. The vestibular organ and *cochlea* (hearing portion of inner ear) together comprise the labyrinth or inner ear.

Semicircular canals: three balance canals (horizontal or lateral, posterior, and superior or anterior) within the inner ear that contain the sensory organs to detect rotational movements in the three dimensions. The *semicircular canals, utricle,* and, *saccule* comprise the five neurosensory elements within the *vestibular organ* or balance organ within the inner ear. The vestibular organ and *cochlea* (hearing portion of inner ear) together comprise the labyrinth or inner ear.

Singular Neurectomy: an operation to cut the *posterior ampullary (singular) nerve.* It is the nerve that sends impulses exclusively from the posterior semicircular canal to the balance part of the brain and may be divided to treat *Benign Paroxysmal Positional Vertigo (BPPV). Particle repositioning maneuvers* or *posterior semicircular canal occlusion* are more commonly used to treat *BPPV.*

Smooth pursuit system: one of the three eye movement control systems to aid the VOR to maintain clear visual imaging of the world when the head moves or a person is seeing objects in motion. The other two eye movement control systems are *optokinetic* and *saccades*. Smooth pursuit is used to follow objects moving slowly across the visual field such as tracking a bird in flight.

Stapes bone (Stirrup): the third and smallest of the three bones in the middle ear. Motion of the stapes is normally responsible for the transmission of sound as mechanical energy into the inner ear.

Stenosis: narrowing of a tubular organ. Atherosclerotic plaque can narrow or even block arteries to the brain, heart, and other organs leading to disease from lack of blood flow.

Streptomycin: one of the *aminoglycoside* antibiotics that may be given as an *intramuscular* (into the muscle) treatment to take advantage of its vestibular toxicity side effects to treat Ménière's disease affecting both inner ears (bilateral *Ménière's disease*).

Stria vascularis: the vascular tissue within the cochlea responsible for producing inner ear fluid called *endolymph*.

Substitution: recovery process in which the brain learns to use the eyes and feet (proprioception) when both inner ear vestibular organs have failed.

Superior Canal Dehiscence Syndrome: a syndrome of vertigo and *oscillopsia* induced by loud noises or by stimuli that change middle ear or intracranial (inside the skull cavity) pressure has recently been defined in patients with a dehiscence (opening) in the bone overlying the superior semicircular canal. These patients may also experience chronic dysequilibrium.

Supine: position of lying-down on one's back.

Sway-referenced vision: whenever you sway forward or back, the visual surroundings will sway with you, but it is inaccurate and not helpful for maintaining your balance. People who are overly dependent on their vision will become very unstable or even fall on this condition that can be reproduced during *dynamic platform posturography.*

Syncope: (pronounced sink-o-pee) an unexpected loss of consciousness.

Temporal bone: the portion of the skull that contains the ear and inner ear.

Tinnitus: abnormal ringing or other noises perceived from the ear or head.

Titrate (Titration): giving small amounts of a medication until reaching a desired effect.

Tonic neck reflex: a stabilizing reflex stimulated by turning the head to a fixed position looking to the right or the left. The arms and legs on the side to which the head is turned extend and ones on the opposite side contract.

Translational motion: linear motion of an object such as the head in side-to-side, front-to-back, up-down, directions.

Tullio phenomenon: vertigo and or eye movements (*nystagmus*) caused by exposure to a loud noise. It is most commonly associated with *Ménière's disease* and *Superior Semicircular Canal Dehiscence Syndrome (SSCD).*

Tympanic cavity: the middle ear. The normally air-filled space behind the eardrum *(tympanic membrane).*

Tympanic membrane: the eardrum

Utricle (Utriculus): One of the five neurosensory organs within the *vestibular organ* that senses linear motion in a forward and backward direction. The 3 *semicircular canals, utricle,* and *saccule,* comprise the five neurosensory elements within the *vestibular organ* or balance organ within the inner ear. The vestibular organ and *cochlea* (hearing portion of inner ear) together comprise the labyrinth or inner ear.

Utricular Macula: sensory epithelium of the utricle responsive to linear accleration especially sensitive to the forces of gravity experienced during head or body tilt.

Vaso-vagal syncope: see neurocardiogenic syncope.

Vascular insufficiency: reduction in blood supply to an organ. It can cause lightheadedness if blood flow is reduced to the brain.

Vertigo: from the Latin verb "to turn;" an hallucination of motion when no motion is actually occurring.

Vestibular Autorotation Test (VAT): a simpler and much less expensive system to measure rotational responses such as the VOR without using a rotational chair. It involves acceleration sensors that are strapped to the head, after which the patient is instructed to rotate the head side to side (or up and down) in time with an increasingly fast clicking sound.

Vestibular Evoked Myogenic Potentials (VEMP): a test that involves the use of loud tones to cause a reflex response in the neck muscles. This response is recorded with electrodes on the skin overlying the muscles. These responses most likely arise from the *sacculus*, one of the vestibular endorgans in the inner ear. VEMP is abnormal in the *Superior Semicircular Canal Dehiscence Syndrome (SSCD).*

Vestibular nerve section (VNS) or vestibular neurectomy: a neurosurgical procedure to sever the vestibular, or balance, nerve. The divided nerve will no longer be able to send "dizzy" signals to the brain.

Vestibular neuritis (or neuronitis): inflammation of the balance or vestibular nerves causing acute vertigo, generally without hearing loss.

Vestibular nuclei: clusters of nerve cells within the brainstem and cerebellum responsible for integrating and processing information concerning all of the balance system including vestibular function, proprioception, and vision.

Vestibular rehabilitation: Vestibular rehabilitation is a term used for exercises that are commonly provided for people with balance and dizziness problems, often administered by physical therapists.

Vestibular suppressants: medications to quiet the balance system and reduce the symptoms of dizziness.

Vestibulo-Ocular Reflex (VOR): functions primarily to stabilize the eyes so that you can continue to see clearly whenever your head is moving. The inner ear senses movement (acceleration) in one direction and the reflex causes your eyes to go in the opposite direction with an equal speed. In that manner your vision is maintained on the original object without becoming blurred. Vestibular testing measures the *gain, phase,* and *asymmetry* of the VOR.

Vestibule or vestibular (end-) organ: the balance organ within the inner ear and comprised of five neurosensory elements. Three of the elements are the semicircular canals that detect rotational motion in the three dimensions of space. One is the utricle that detects linear motion in a forward and backward direction. One is the saccule that detects linear motion in an upward and downward direction.

Vestibulo-spinal tracts: nerve fibers descending from vestibular nuclei in the brainstem into the spinal cord. They participate in reflexes important for maintaining balance and posture.

Videonystagmography: vestibular testing employing infrared camera goggles to keep the subject's vision dark and suppress the natural reflex for focusing on an object to suppress nystagmus but still allowing video recording of eye movements.

Visual fixation suppression: natural response to suppress even fairly strong nystagmus and vertigo by staring at a fixed object. Staring at the horizon can help motion sickness to pass and staring at a fixed spot helps prevent vertigo during pirouettes.

VOR: see Vestibulo-Ocular Reflex

Bibliography

Headache Classification Committee of the International Headache Society. Classification and diagnostic criteria for headache disorders, cranial neuralgias and facial pain. Cephalgia 1988; 8:19-73.

Johnson GD, Medical Management of Migraine-Related Dizziness and Vertigo. Laryngoscope 1998;108 Supplement 85:1-28.

Index